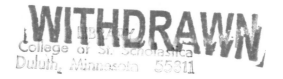

AGING
AND
INCOME

Aging Series

Long-Term Care of Older People
Brody, E., M.S.W.

Retirement
Carp, F. M., Ph.D.

Time, Roles, and Self in Old Age
Gubrium, J. F., Ph.D.

Aging and Income: Programs and Prospects for the Elderl
Herzog, B. R., Ph.D. (ed.)

Toward a Theology of Aging
Hiltner, S., Th.D.

Research, Planning, and Action for the Elderly
Kent, D. P., Ph.D., Kastenbaum, R., Ph.D., and Sherwood, S., Ph.D.

Sound Sex and the Aging Heart
Scheingold, L. D., M.A., and Wagner, N., Ph.D.

Counseling Older Persons
Sinick D., Ph.D.

On Dying and Denying
Weisman, A., M.D.

The Gerontological Apperception Test
Wolk, R. L., Ph.D and Wolk, R. B., Ph.D.

Edited by Barbara Rieman Herzog

AGING
AND
INCOME

Programs and Prospects for the Elderly

Special Publication No. 4
Sponsored by
the Gerontological Society

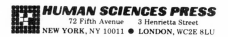 **HUMAN SCIENCES PRESS**
72 Fifth Avenue   3 Henrietta Street
NEW YORK, NY 10011 ● LONDON, WC2E 8LU

Library of Congress Catalog Number 78-2510

ISBN: 0-87705-369-3

Copyright © 1978 by Human Sciences Press 72 Fifth Avenue, New York, New York 10011

Printed in the United States of America
89 987654321

Library of Congress Cataloging in Publication Data

Main entry under title:

Aging and income.

   (Special publication sponsored by the Gerontological Society ; no. 4)
   Includes bibliographies and index.
   1. Old age assistance—United States—Addresses, essays, lectures. 2. Retirement income—United States—Addresses, essays, lectures. 3. Aged—United States—Economic conditions—Addresses, essays, lectures.
I. Herzog, Barbara Rieman. II. Series: Gerontological Society. Special publication sponsored by the Gerontological Society ; no. 4.
HV1461.A52 362.6'0973   78-2510

CONTENTS

CONTRIBUTORS

Esther Ammundsen, M.D., received her medical degree from Copenhagen University in 1939, and a degree in public health in 1940. Following World War II she was involved in hospital and relief work, and in 1951 she became Commissioner of Health for the City of Copenhagen. In 1962 Dr. Ammundsen was named Denmark's Director General of Health. She held the post until 1974, when she became a consultant to the Copenhagen regional office of the World Health Organization.

R. Meredith Belbin, Ph.D., is an industrial training consultant whose academic career at the University of Cambridge, England, took him from classics through psychology to gerontology. After receiving a doctorate for his thesis on the employment of older workers in industry, he moved into engineering production and worked in a wide range of industries. In recent years his activities on behalf of the Organization for Economic Cooperation and Development (OECD) have included setting up demonstration projects on the training of older workers in Austria, Sweden, the U.K., and the U.S.A. He currently has appointments to the Commission of the European Communities, the Industrial Training Research Unit at Cambridge, and the Administrative Staff College at Henley, England. He is also working as adviser to several industrial corporations.

Robert C. Benedict, M.P.A., has been nominated as national Commissioner on Aging, having previously served as Commissioner of the Office for the Aging of Pennsylvania. Before assuming this position in 1972, he was Director of Short-Term Training and the Residential Institute on Aging of the Institute of Gerontology at the University of Michigan/Wayne State University in Ann Arbor. He is the author of a number of articles and reports on services for the elderly.

Henry P. Brehm, Ph.D., currently holds the position of Adjunct Associate Professor of Sociology at the University of Maryland. He serves as Associate Editor of the *Journal of Health and Social Behavior,* and has been a Guest Editor of the *Milbank Memorial Fund Quarterly/Health and Society.* Dr. Brehm is the author (with Rodney M. Coe) of *Preventive Health Care for Adults,* and is currently interested in the future of health care delivery in the United States.

Robert L. Clark, Ph.D., is a Senior Fellow of the Center for the Study of Aging and Human Development at Duke University and Assistant Professor of Economics and Business at North Carolina State University. Dr. Clark's current research interests center around the future costs of dependency programs, life cycle patterns of saving and consumption, and mobility patterns of older workers. He is the author (with Juanita Kreps) of *Sex, Age and Work: The Changing Composition of the Labor Force,* and is currently preparing a study of the role of private pensions in maintaining retirement income for the National Planning Association.

Robert J. Havighurst, Ph.D., is Professor of Education and Human Development at the University of Chicago. He has served as President of the Gerontological Society and has received the

Kleemeier Award for outstanding research in the field of gerontology. During 1974–1975 he coordinated the interdisciplinary
Project on the Future of Aging at the University of Chicago. Dr.
Havighurst is the author or editor of many books in the fields of
education and gerontology, most recently *Social Policy, Social Ethics and the Aging Society* (with Bernice L. Neugarten). He is currently interested in the sociology of aging and the effects of
energy shortages on the participation of elderly workers in the
labor force.

Barbara Rieman Herzog, Ph.D. (Editor) served as a grant project
director for the Gerontological Society from 1970 to 1976. She
arranged for the preparation of the chapters which comprise this
book, and planned an April 1976 Conference on Support for the
Elderly, which was based on material presented in these chapters.
Before that she served as a research analyst for the Department
of State, where she authored many reports on China and North
Vietnam and on U.S. Far Eastern policy. Ms. Herzog is currently
Special Assistant to the Executive Director of the National
Retired Teachers Association/American Association of Retired
Persons.

Francis P. King, Ph.D., is the Senior Research Officer of the Teachers Insurance and Annuity Association and College Retirement
Equities Fund. In this capacity he is responsible for surveys and
studies of insurance and retirement benefit plans in the field of
higher education, and he is the author of a number of books and
articles in this field. He is coauthor (with Dr. William C. Green-
ough) of *Pension Plans and Public Policy,* which was published in
1976 by Columbia University Press under a grant from the Ford
Foundation. He also serves as Chairman of the Board of Tuition
Exchange, Inc.

Malcolm H. Morrison, Ph.D., is Adjunct Professor of Social Gerontology at Antioch College, Columbia, Maryland. He received his
doctorate in 1974 from the Florence Heller School of Brandeis
University, where he specialized in the economics of aging. Dr.

Morrison's interests center on the economic, social, and psychological aspects of retirement. His past publications have been concerned with the economic behavior of workers in planning for retirement. At present he is examining human relations problem-solving approaches for older workers and is engaged in research for a book on flexible retirement.

Alicia Haydock Munnell, Ph.D., is an Assistant Vice-President and Economist at the Federal Reserve Bank of Boston. She began developing her expertise on the Social Security System while at the Brookings Institution in Washington, D.C. In 1972 the Social Security Administration awarded Harvard University a research grant based on Dr. Munnell's proposal to explore the impact of the Social Security program on individuals' savings behavior. *The Effect of Social Security on Personal Saving* summarizes the results of that study. She has recently finished another book, *The Future of Social Security*, which discusses alternatives for the overall reform of the program.

Joseph J. Spengler, Ph.D., is the James B. Duke Professor of Economics, Emeritus, at Duke University. He has been president of many learned societies, including the American Economic Association (1965) and more recently the History of Economics Society and the Atlantic Economic Society. Dr. Spengler is the author of numerous books and articles in the field of individual and population aging. He is currently working on a book about the economics of a stationary population.

PREFACE

The chapters in this book were commissioned in early 1976, at a time when the American public was becoming seriously concerned about demographic change and about how the large numbers of future elderly will be supported.

The rate of increase in the older population has indeed been great in the last 25 years, and it is not surprising that the press and the public have begun to pay attention to demographic projections. What is not generally understood, however, is that the rate of growth is likely to be relatively slow in the next quarter century, only to rise again very sharply after the year 2010. Thus during the next quarter century we have a breather—time to establish the policies which will have such an impact when the retiree bulge finally occurs between 2010 and 2040.

The various chapters in this book offer predictions of the future and suggest choices for continuity or change. Among the areas discussed are the characteristics and needs of the future elderly; the total costs to the working population of supporting the dependent population, both old and young; the impact of our energy choices on the elderly; the best mix of private pensions and Social Security; how public support payments should be made; how monies to finance such payments should be collected; and methods of providing income-in-kind in the form of health care and social services.

The question of how much work-generated income the future elderly will have is central to devising appropriate public support policies. Are we to promote increasingly earlier retirement and larger support burdens? Or are there policies which might offer the elderly a greater choice in their allocation of time between leisure, education, and work, and which would enhance their quality of life at minimal or no expense to the public treasury? How difficult would it really be to spread out the working life somewhat longer? Would people be willing to work (at least part-time) more years into late adulthood in return for more flexibility in allocating their time during their earlier working years?

Because of the need to reexamine Social Security financing, we can expect continued interest in the question of public support for the elderly. Efforts must be made to ensure that all older people have a livable income. There would be much merit, however, in going beyond this goal and examining how to provide greater opportunities for choice between work, education, and leisure so as to enhance the overall quality of life for adults of all ages.

The contents of these chapters were first discussed by a small group of government, academic, business, and labor leaders who met in April 1976 under the aegis of the Gerontological Society, with the support of the Administration of Aging. The conference was chaired by William Bechill, former U.S. Commissioner on Aging.

This volume is the fourth in a series of Special Publications sponsored by the Gerontological Society under the overall guidance of M. Powell Lawton, Editor-in-Chief, and Mary Wylie, Editor for Social Research, Planning and Practice, whose efforts contributed greatly to its quality.

Barbara Rieman Herzog

-Part I-

THE SETTING: ANTICIPATED DEMOGRAPHIC AND SOCIAL CHANGE

As background for the other articles in this collection, gerontologist Robert J. Havighurst examines the status, needs, and wants of the future elderly. He predicts that the near future (to 1990) is likely to be a rather stable period, except for the uncertainties resulting from monetary inflation.

In contrast, the intermediate future (1990–2030) could be very unstable. In Havighurst's view, the costs of energy will control the socioeconomic structure of the 21st century, and those costs are likely to keep climbing. High energy costs will be compounded by high prices for scarce materials, resulting in substantial downward pressures on the material standard of living. People will probably respond by working more years or longer hours to increase production and maintain their present standards, and the elderly will be encouraged to remain in the labor force longer.

One concomitant may be additional emphasis on skills testing and retraining. Another may be lower Social Security taxes and smaller pension trust funds. High energy costs may even affect living arrangements: Havighurst foresees the creation of colonies located on the outskirts of big cities, where the elderly could raise enough food to be partially self-supporting, while still having access by public transportation to family and friends, as well as to the theaters, libraries, and churches of the city.

In making his predictions, Havighurst envisions an economy which, though beset by higher energy costs, will be healthy enough to provide employment for all the people who he assumes will want to work harder to maintain their standard of living. He does not address the possibility of high unemployment and a low rate of growth, and the resulting effects of this constellation on his predictions of greater participation in the labor force by the elderly, and lower Social Security and pension costs.

In the subsequent article, economists Joseph Spengler and Robert Clark explain the demographic changes which are likely to occur during the next 75 years. They note, as have others, that although fewer working people will be called upon to support more old people, the total dependency ratio will not increase during the next 75 years. Spengler and Clark then address the difficult question of whether—assuming current levels of public expenditure per old person and per child are maintained—working people will be paying out more or fewer tax dollars to support the dependents of the future. The answer to this question has clear implications for an issue which worries many people: whether the nation will be able to "afford" to continue or to increase its support for the elderly. On the basis of their model, the authors conclude that total dependency costs as a percentage of disposable personal income will decline very slightly after 2000, whereupon they will rise again until, in 2050, they are two percentage points higher than today. Whether this increase is considered small or large lies very much in the eye of the beholder.

Spengler and Clark are cognizant of the difficulties of their task. They point out, for example, that they may be assuming too high a level of disposable personal income, since expenditures on older people do not have the same positive effect on economic growth as expenditures on youth. If personal income were lower, the effective dependency burden would be higher. They also note that tax dollars saved because there will be fewer children cannot necessarily be shifted to the support of increased numbers of older people. Voters may resist this shift, preferring instead to increase expenditures per child.

The authors emphasize they are not passing moral judgments: support for the elderly is not "better" than support for children (or vice versa), nor are payments for children's education qualitatively the same as Social Security retirement benefits.

Their conclusions can at best point in a general direction: costs will be greater. How much greater is not clear at this point, because they have not yet included in their model the amount which states and localities contribute to welfare and health programs such as Medicaid. (Inclusion would add to the projected cost increase, but it is premature to say by how much.)

Factors which are beyond the scope of their paper may have an important impact on what level of overall costs workers will be willing to support. The authors touch only briefly on the impact of *private* dependency costs. Since such costs per child are far greater than per older person, future demographic change may reduce the overall private burden, even as the public burden is increasing.

Finally, how easily a given burden is managed is a function of the state of the economy, and this too is beyond the scope of Clark and Spengler's study. If productivity and personal income are increasing rapidly, the same dependency costs will be relatively lighter. However, if productivity is not increasing and high unemployment also exists, costs will be relatively heavier, and the pool of workers bearing those costs will be smaller. The health of the economy will thus have a significant impact on the political viability of increased support for the elderly.

-1-

Social Change: The Status, Needs, and Wants of the Future Elderly

Robert J. Havighurst

The purpose of this essay is to examine the social and personal situation of the elderly population and their needs and wants, with major attention to the future. The future will be divided into two segments: the near future, 1978–1990, and the intermediate future, 1990–2030.

The near future is quite clearly visible, and we already know pretty well what the needs and wants of the elderly will be in the next 12 years. But the intermediate future is obscure, partly because it will depend on socioeconomic developments and policies to be made in the near future, and partly because it depends on at least two things about which we cannot be sure even in 1990 —the supply and cost of energy and essential materials, and the economic-political relations of the United States with other nations.

We may look first at the near future, and then in a more speculative but important mode at the intermediate future.

THE NEAR FUTURE—1978–1990

The next 12 years, from 1978 to 1990, will see little change in the relative size of the elderly population, as can be noted in Table 1.1. Between now and the end of the century, the popula-

Table 1.1 Demographic Projections, 1975–2050

Age Group	Numbers in Millions				
	1975	1990	2000	2025	2050
Under 20	74.6	74.9	79.2	83.2	87.5
15 – 24	40.2	34.8	38.8	40.9	43.3
20 – 64	116.6	141.3	152.6	168.4	179.7
55+	42.1	49.4	53.5	82.2	87.4
65+	22.3	28.9	30.6	48.1	51.2
75+	8.4	11.4	13.5	18.0	22.1
Total	213.5	245.1	262.5	299.7	318.4

Percent under 20	35.0	30.6	30.1	27.7	27.4
Percent 65+	10.4	11.8	11.7	16.0	16.1
Percent 75+	3.9	4.7	5.1	6.0	6.9
Percent 20-64	54.5	57.7	58.1	56.1	56.5
Percent 65-74	6.5	7.1	6.5	10.0	9.2
Ratio under 20:20-64	.64	.53	.52	.50	.49
Ratio 65+:20-64	.19	.20	.20	.29	.28

Source: U.S. Bureau of the Census, (1975, Tables 8 and 11, Series II).

tion aged 65 and over will increase from 10.4 to 11.7 percent of the total population—a very modest increase. This projection is based upon the assumption that fertility in the United States will be at 2.11 (approximately the replacement level) during the next 25 years, and that there will be a net immigration of about 400,000 persons per year. The projection also assumes a slight reduction in mortality rates, which will add about two years to life expectancy at age 65.

Parenthetically, it is amazing how inept many people are when it comes to naming the proportions of the elderly population. In the Harris Poll of 1974 (National Council on the Aging, 1975), a national sample of adults was asked what proportion of the population is over 65 years of age, and the most frequent answer was "between 30 and 39 percent." And in a hearing before the Special Committee on Aging of the United States Senate, on June 30, 1975, a member of the state board of psychological examiners in New Jersey, who introduced herself as a "psychologist and sociologist" said, "I wish to give you an estimate that in the year 2000, it is projected that half of the population of this country will be age 65 and over." The cover story in *Time Magazine* on June 2, 1975, announced that the over-65 population in the year 2000 would amount to 20 percent of the total population.

Economic Welfare.   We cannot be so certain about the future economic welfare of the elderly, because our economy has experienced a great deal of monetary inflation since 1970. Inflation reduces the real income of people living on a fixed dollar income, as elderly people tend to do, except for their social security benefits, which since 1972 have been raised as the cost of living increased. (However it should be noted that many elderly people own their homes and therefore are protected against the inflationary rise in housing costs.) The median income for an elderly household was about $5,000 in the summer of 1974, according to the Harris Poll of the population over 65 which was taken at that time. The "poverty level" income, as defined by the federal government for a nonfarm individual aged 65 or over was $2,364, and for an elderly couple, $2,982. At that time approximately 16 percent of the elderly population were below those levels. In the 1974 Harris Poll, 15 percent of the national sample stated that "not having enough money to live on" was a "very serious problem."

If we count the 16 percent of elderly persons below the poverty level in 1974 and add another 9 percent who are not more than $700 above the poverty line and may be thought of as "near poor," we get about 5.5 million elderly persons or one in four who have a major income problem. The federal government system of Supplemental Security Income provides funds to raise the minimum annual income of a single person to $1,750 and to $2,500 for a couple, both well below the official poverty level.

Obviously the economic status of 25 percent of the elderly population is far from satisfactory, and the present system of Supplemental Security Income does not lift the income of poor people even to the official poverty level.

A retirement income or replacement income of about 70 percent of the previous wage or salary income will support an elderly person who is in good health at a level roughly comparable to what he had attained while he was employed. This might well be defined as a need of all retired persons, and therefore a reasonable goal for Social Security benefits. The Western European countries do provide about this level of retirement benefits through their old age pension plans. But an American worker who earned the federal minimum wage in his last year before retirement would, if single, receive Social Security payments of 62 percent of that amount, and a worker who earned the maximum covered amount in 1975 ($13,000) would receive Social Security benefits of 31 percent of that amount. If a married man retired at age 65 with median level earnings, he and his wife would receive Social Security payments amounting to 65 percent of the amount of his final earnings.

It is true, of course, that many Americans also receive pensions from private employers and that many others have annuity income from savings they have made and to which their employers may have contributed.

A generous estimate would be that three-quarters of elderly people have incomes adequate enough to maintain the material standard of living to which they have been accustomed. The principal economic problem for them is the danger of continued

monetary inflation at more than a two or three percent increase
in the cost of living per year. This is one area which needs research and governmental action in the immediate future.

Problems and Needs. To get a general overview of the needs
and problems of the elderly, we can turn to a 1974 Harris Poll
(National Council on the Aging, 1975). The sample of elderly
people was enlarged for this particular poll, as was the sample of
blacks, to provide more reliable data than would otherwise have
been possible. The respondents were shown a list of possible
problems and asked how serious each was for them personally,
and how serious they thought each problem was for "most people over 65." Possible responses were "very serious," "somewhat
serious," "hardly a problem at all," and "not sure." Table 1.2
reports the responses, broken down for the personal problems
by the educational level of the respondent.

The two problems which received the highest number of "very
serious" mentions were "fear of crime" and "poor health," followed by a middle group consisting of "not enough money,"
"loneliness," "not enough medical care," "not enough education," and "not feeling needed." With the exception of "fear of
crime," the problems fall into the familiar categories of employment and income, health services, and social interaction.

Employment and Labor Force Participation. The 20th century has a history of reduced employment among elderly men,
with some increased employment among elderly women. In
1900, two-thirds of the men over 65 were employed; now less
than one-fourth are working for money. For men in the age range
65–69, 59 percent were employed in 1940 and 33 percent were
employed in 1975. The employment of elderly women has increased, from 9 percent for those aged 65–69 in 1940, to 15
percent in 1975.

The change for men is mainly due to the voluntary retirement
of men who become eligible for Social Security or pension benefits. Mandatory retirement at a fixed age is a factor, but not the
major factor.

The forces which control the employment of older men and
women are primarily economic ones, although the individual's

own attitude toward work and, of course, the individual's health, are important in his individual action. The economic forces work as follows:

1. The individual's need of income tends to determine his participation.
2. The economy's need for workers tends to determine the state of the labor market for older workers.
3. The relation between Social Security benefits and remuneration from employment tends to determine the elderly individual's decision about seeking employment. Table 1.3 summarizes the data on labor force participation since 1950.

Two other factors affect the employment of elderly people: (1) the Age Discrimination Act, which bans discrimination in employment because of age up to age 65. If this act were to be amended to raise the age limit to 70 or 75, it would increase the employment of persons in those age brackets, but probably only to a limited degree. (2) Provisions for changing work assignments so as to match jobs with personal skills and abilities after age 55 or 60. The best known example is the program instituted by Dr. Leon Koyl of the DeHavilland Aircraft Corporation in Canada, and applied in a major demonstration experiment supported by the U.S. Department of Labor in Portland, Maine. Employees may take a battery of seven tests to measure their physical and mental abilities, and they may then be shifted to different jobs whose profiles of needed abilities match the individuals' personal profiles.

THE NEXT 12 YEARS. The economic recession which struck the American economy at the end of 1973 is not fully reflected in Table 1.4, which reports official unemployment figures in 1974. The overall unemployment rate went up to about eight percent in 1975, then began to drop as economic activity increased.

The employment rate of men and women aged 55 to 75 is likely to remain stable at the present level through 1978–1990. In spite of the real problem of holding a job experienced by a minority of workers in their 50s, the unemployment rates are relatively

Table 1.2 "Very Serious" Problems for People Over 65 (Percent of National Sample, 65 and Over)

| Problem | Felt Personally | | | | Attributed to "Most People over 65" by People over 65 |
	Total Group	Educational Level A	B	C	
Fear of crime	23	25	23	10	51
Poor health	21	26	14	9	53
Not having enough money to live on	15	20	8	3	59
Loneliness	12	15	9	6	56
Not enough medical care	10	13	5	5	36
Not enough education	8	12	2	1	25

Not feeling needed	7	9	5	2	40
Not enough to do to keep busy	6	7	4	2	33
Not enough friends	5	5	3	2	26
Not enough job opportunities	5	7	3	4	32
Poor housing	4	5	2	1	34
Not enough clothing	3	4	1	-	17

Highest Educational Level of Respondent: A Some High School or Less
                                                     B High School Graduate or Some College
                                                     C College Graduate

Source: Reprinted from *The Myth and Reality of Aging in America*, a study prepared by Louis Harris and Associates, Inc., for the National Council on Aging, Inc., Washington, DC, 1975, p. 36.

Table 1.3 Labor Force Participation Rates, 1950–1975

	Percent in Labor Force					
	1950	1960	1965	1970	1975
All males					
55-64	87	88	85	83	76
55-59	NA	92	90	90	84
59-64	NA	82	78	75	66
65+	46	33	28	26	22
65-69		47	43	39	32
70+		25	19	17	15
Non-white males					
55-64	82	83	79	79	69
55-59	NA	NA	NA	84	77
60-64	NA	NA	NA	74	59
65+	46	31	28	27	20.9
65-69	NA	NA	NA	NA	NA
70+	NA	NA	NA	NA	NA

26

All females					
55–64	27	38	41	43	41
55–59	NA	45	47	49	48
60–64	NA	31	34	36	33
65+	9.8	11.9	10.0	9.7	8.3
65–69	NA	19.0	17.4	17.3	14.5
70+	NA	7.8	6.1	5.7	4.9
Non-white females					
55–64	49	47	49	47	44
55–59	NA	NA	NA	53	52
60–64	NA	NA	NA	39	35
65+	16.5	12.8	12.9	12.2	10.5
65–69	NA	NA	NA	NA	NA
70+	NA	NA	NA	NA	NA

Source: U.S. Bureau of the Census, (1976, Table 6–5).

Table 1.4 Unemployment in Relation to Age and Sex, 1974

Age	Unemployment rate (Percent of Civilian Labor Force)	
	Male	Female
16-19	15.5	16.5
20-24	8.7	9.5
25-44	3.2	5.4
45-54	2.4	3.3
55-64	2.6	3.3
65 plus	3.3	3.7
National Unemployment Rate	4.8	6.7

Source: U.S. Department of Labor (1975, Table 6).

lower for the 55–64 age group than for the younger groups. This rate depends on the answers given by a sample of people to a government survey question asking whether they are unemployed and seeking work. There are others who say they are not seeking work. However, some of them would accept a job if it were offered to them.

The age group 55–75 is not going to change appreciably in relative size during the remainder of this century. It will stay at about 15 percent of the total population, while the 20–55 group will increase in proportion and will probably experience more difficulty in the job market for that reason. Although the 20–55 group will compete with those over-55 for jobs, it seems likely that the over-55 group will hold their jobs fairly steadily, because they will have the advantage of seniority.

The conditions which will determine the employment level of the elderly will be the following:

- The demand for workers.
- The purchasing power of retirement incomes.
- The attitudes of older workers toward their jobs.
- The laws and practices concerning mandatory retirement.
- Government policies and programs of employment for older workers.

Assuming that the economy recovers fairly soon and then grows slowly for the remainder of this century, it seems likely that the over-55 population will be employed at about the level they had reached in 1970. Even if retirement incomes should improve for many people, senior citizens are a work-centered group and are likely to hold on to their jobs much as they do today. The attitudes of older workers are fairly favorable toward their jobs, despite rumors to the contrary. Thus the longitudinal study of middle-aged men in the labor force being conducted by Parnes and his colleagues at Ohio State University reports that workers aged 60 to 64 were more favorable toward their jobs than were men aged 50 to 59. For the years 1966, 1969, and 1971, the proportions of white men aged 60–64 who said that they liked their jobs "very much" were 68, 62, and 51 respectively, while only four to five percent said they disliked their jobs. The remainder liked their jobs "somewhat." True, there was a decline in the proportion of those who reported liking their jobs "very much," but the vote was still very positive and does not indicate that men in their 50s and 60s are likely to leave the labor market by free choice (Parnes, 1974).

This rather optimistic view of the position of older workers in the labor force does not mean that the existing efforts to increase and maintain employment of older workers are unnecessary or undesirable. Such efforts and programs probably serve to keep the pressure on employers and government to provide work and earnings for a substantial marginal group of elderly persons. The Illinois Department of Aging recently listed the following efforts to provide income-earning opportunities (U.S. Senate Special Committee on Aging, 1975).

- Encouragement of employers to utilize elderly workers who can be hired in a number of part-time jobs.
- Increasing emphasis on human services roles for elderly workers.
- Increased sponsorship of sheltered workshops utilizing subcontract operations from industry and employing both aging and elderly workers.
- Creation of specialized "case finding," referral, and placement of elderly persons utilizing elderly volunteers and elderly placement personnel in major roles.
- Special training programs to assist both aging and elderly persons to achieve opportunities in new careers to increase their employment alternatives.
- Encouragement of self-employment of elderly persons as free-lance entrepreneurs.

Living Arrangements. Generally speaking, living arrangements include regional geographical location, urban-rural location, and types of housing. There are four generalizations about the living arrangements of elderly people which are supported by the data in Table 1.5.

1. Older married couples prefer to live independently of their adult children, but within easy reach of them. The Harris Poll of 1974 found that 81 percent of the elderly people who have living children have seen some of their children "within the last week or so." But only about nine percent of people over 65 actually lived in the household of an adult child.

2. There are two general forms of migration of older people. One is to the "retirement states" of Florida, Arizona, and California. In the 1965–1970 period, about three percent of the people over 65 moved from one state to another that was not contiguous. Nearly all of these moves were to the three states just mentioned. The other migration is from small towns and cities to larger cities or metropolitan areas. In the 1965–1970 period, one percent of the people over 65 moved from a small town or city into a metropolitan area.

3. The proportion of elderly persons living in urbanized metropolitan areas increased from about 44 percent in 1950 to 55 percent in 1970. This was largely due to the earlier migration of younger people into metropolitan areas, who then remained there as they grew older. The geographer Stephen Golant (1975) has pointed out that an adult population tends to remain "in place" as they grow older, unless there are major forces to cause them to move, such as physical deterioration of a neighborhood or ethnic migrations. Thus the elderly may be left behind when younger adults move to suburbs. Golant expects that by the year 2000 a larger proportion of the total American elderly population will be located in metropolitan areas.

4. Although low-rent public housing designed for the elderly is presently insufficient to meet the existing demand, over the last 15 years this form of accommodation has experienced a remarkable growth. In 1960 there were just over 18,000 dwelling units designed for the elderly developed by local housing authorities in contrast to almost 350,000

Table 1.5 Living Arrangements of Older Persons, 1970 (Percentages)

	55–64	65–74	65+	75+
Marital status				
Men: married, wife present	82	75		56
widowed	4	11		28
Women: married, husband present	64	44		19
widowed	20	42		68
Urban-rural location				
Urbanized areas (50,000+)	58	56		55
Other urban (2,500–50,000)	15	17		19
Rural (under 2,500)	27	27		27
Living arrangements				
Men: heads of household	95	93		86
with child/other relative	–	3		12
alone	–	?	14	?
institutions	1	2		7

Women:			
heads of household	27	42	51
with child/other relative	–	11	22
alone	–	?	?
institutions	1	2	11
Of those who had children or grandchildren:			
saw child within last day		34	
or last week			81
saw grandchild within last day			
or last week			75

Source: U.S. Bureau of the Census, (1976, Table 6–2).

in 1972. In the same period Section 202 (nonprofit-sponsored) elderly housing increased from 200 units to over 46,000 units.

Bild and Havighurst (1976) reported some comparative data on the elderly in big cities of various countries and stated the following conclusions:

1. The elderly tend to be somewhat segregated in certain areas of large cities.

2. Every large city has a growing number of elderly immigrants who came to the city from other countries or from other regions of the country as young adults or as children. These immigrants may be different in skin color and in national background from the dominant population in the city.

   Thus the elderly immigrants in Chicago are blacks from the South and Chicanos from the Southwest and Mexico. In London a substantial group of immigrants are from the British West Indies, Pakistan, and Uganda. In New York the most recent immigrants are Southern blacks and Puerto Ricans, and their proportions of elderly are increasing.

3. There are several patterns of independent residence of the elderly in large cities: (a) husband-wife residence in small separate dwelling units; (b) husband-wife residence in large apartment complexes; (c) lone person residence in large apartment complexes; (d) lone person residence in separate dwelling units (declining); (e) lone person residence in rooming houses and residential hotels (growing); (f) lone person residence in homes for the aged (stable, not growing).

A striking fact is the increase of lone persons living in rooming houses and residential hotels, especially in the larger cities. The initials SRO (single room occupancy) have come into common use to designate this arrangement, which has been furthered by the quasi-obsolescence of former luxury hotels and apartment houses in big city areas that are no longer especially fashionable. The people who live in these rooms or small apartments are mainly widows or widowers. They range in economic status from the wealthy to the poor. The residential hotels range from high-status luxury hotels to buildings which accommodate people on incomes just above the poverty level. Viewing these facts and projecting into the near future, Golant (1975, p. 22) has made the following predictions:

1. A higher proportion of the elderly population will be concentrated in metropolitan agglomerations, primarily as a function of natural increases in numbers.

2. "Retirement states" with warm or temperate year-round climates will experience significant economic growth in both their metropolitan and nonmetropolitan centers. This will facilitate the growth of new planned retirement centers and new age-integrated communities, with both housing and services catering to the needs of older persons. However the percentage of American elderly population occupying these communities will continue to be small.

3. The older population living in metropolitan areas will be spatially dispersed over an increasingly large suburban area. Technological advances in transportation and electronic communications will result in geographical distance becoming a less accurate predictor of the frequency or intensity of interpersonal or interneighborhood interactions.

4. An increasing proportion of the elderly in central cities will be black. Thus the white elderly population will become increasingly dispersed throughout the surburban areas and the black elderly increasingly concentrated in central cities. At the same time an increasing number of black communities with relatively high concentrations of elderly will occupy suburban locations outside the central city.

5. The number of neighborhoods and housing structures with relatively high concentrations of elderly persons will increase by the year 2000. A small number of these natural communities will contain an almost all-elderly population living within an infrastructure of housing and services primarily oriented to their needs. In the main, however, age-integrated neighborhoods containing persons in all stages

of the life cycle, occupying a diverse array of housing structures, are likely to predominate.

6. The growth of multifamily "public housing" projects designed for age-segregated elderly persons will continue. These will assume an increasingly more complex set of roles enabling all but the most physically and mentally frail older person to remain in the community, and thus delay institutionalization.

RESEARCH NEEDS. Most of the changes projected in this section are continuations of present trends and do not promise to be drastic or disturbing to the lives of most elderly people. However there is reason to be concerned about the increasing proportions of elderly people who are living alone, on the margin of poverty, in residential hotels and rooming houses. The study of single room occupancy residents made by Bild and Havighurst (1976) in Chicago indicated that those with relatively low incomes had a high incidence of problems, and they had low scores on a Life Satisfaction Inventory. Some qualitative evidence indicates that similar groups are increasing in size in other large cities: London, Paris, New York, and Chicago are all cited by Havighurst as cities in which 25 to 40 percent of the over-65 population live alone. Many of these people have adequate incomes and live quite comfortably, but the subgroup with low incomes is a problem group and might well be studied in several large cities.

SOCIAL RELATIONS. Social relations consist of activity in the roles of spouse, parent, grandparent, neighbor, association member, and friend. The amount of time and energy used in one or another role changes from one period in the life span to another. The changes are likely to be rather sharp and rather stressful in the age period from about 60 to 75 because death of a spouse, retirement from a job, and change of residence often occur, and they force a change in social relations.

FAMILY RELATIONS. The family is a strong and supportive institution for older people, but it differs substantially in its structure and functions for men as compared to women. Because men tend to marry younger women, and because men tend to die younger than women, there is a large discrepancy between the number of widows and the number of widowers. In 1971, 70 percent of men aged 65 and over were living with their wives, 17 percent were widowed, and 13 percent were never married or were divorced or separated. At the same time only 35 percent of women aged 65 and over were living with their husbands, while 54 percent were widowed, and 11 percent were never married or were divorced or separated. A growing number of men and women lived alone in houses or apartments, 15 percent of the men and 36 percent of the women. About seven percent of elderly men and 24 percent of elderly women lived with other relatives, usually with adult children.

Older couples prefer to live in households separate from their adult children, for as long as the couple is together. A national sample of people over 65, in the Harris Poll of 1974, reported on their contacts with children and grandchildren. Eighty-one percent have living children, and 81 percent of this group had seen one or more of their children "within the last week or so," including 55 percent who had seen children within the day. Seventy-five percent had living grandchildren, and 73 percent of this group had seen grandchildren "within the last week or so."

ASSOCIATIONS AND SENIOR CENTERS.   Churches and synagogues are especially important to elderly people. In the 1974 Harris Poll, 79 percent of the people aged 65 and over said they had attended a church or synagogue "within the last week or two," and 71 percent said religion was "very important" in their lives. For many elderly people, the church or synagogue is both a place of worship and a place of association with friends.

Senior centers are less widespread, of course, but 51 percent in the 65 and over group said there was a senior citizens' center or golden age club convenient for them to attend. About one-third of this group (18 percent of the 65 and over group) reported that they had attended a golden age club or senior citizens' center within the past year, and two-thirds of this one third had attended within the last month.

INFORMAL SOCIAL RELATIONS.   The informal social relations consist of relations with friends, neighbors, and colleagues or acquaintances. These relations tend to become more important to people as they grow older and retire from their worker role, and as they have more time on their hands.

In a study of retired male teachers and industrial workers in five European and American metropolitan areas, Havighurst and deVries (1969) found five patterns of informal social relations, which are listed in Table 1.6.

IMPLICATIONS FOR THE FUTURE. While these patterns of social relations will probably persist with little change during the next 12 years, the slowly growing concentration of elderly people in certain neighborhoods of big cities and in retirement communities should be monitored, to find out what patterns of social relations are the most satisfactory to various groups of elderly people. For instance, the rapid growth of senior centers and of clubs and informal senior social groups should be studied to find out whether the trend toward age-segregated social relations represented by these developments is proving to be generally valuable. It is probable that a minority of older people will deliberately avoid age-segregated activities, at least while they are in the young old-age period of 55 to 75.

Civic-Political Action. There is a good deal of guessing about the future political attitudes and actions of the elderly population. It is known that people over 60 are more likely than are young adults to vote in most elections. If the elderly were to form a voting bloc, they could certainly exert a large amount of pressure on the government. They might be able to vote solidly on certain issues that affect senior citizens most directly. But there is no evidence that the elderly population votes on national issues differently from the way they did when they were 20 or 30 years younger. Thus it is not likely that the majority of elders will vote as a bloc for one or another party in a national election.

However there have been and will continue to be pervasive political consequences resulting from the age structure of the American population. A special issue of *The Annals* entitled *Political Consequences of Aging* gives a broad overview and raises a variety of questions about probable political developments which indicate the need for more research and for continued monitoring of

Table 1.6 Patterns of Informal Social Relations (Percentages)

	Teachers	Industrial Workers
Replaces old with new social relations, without reducing activity in this area	24	8
Sticks to old relationships, with little or no reduction of activity	20	41
Withdraws slowly from relations with other people	44	37
Cuts himself off from former relations and does not make new ones.	8	8
A "loner": never had close friends or other associates	4	6

Source: Havighurst & deVries (1969). Reprinted with permission of S. Karger AG, Basel, Switzerland.

the impact of the situation of the elderly on the American political scene.

The several writers of articles in *The Annals* are not in basic disagreement, but they stress different aspects. Robert Binstock (1974) sees the political conscience of the society becoming more and more concerned with the needs of the elderly, but he observes little or no effective use of "senior power" in politics. But Henry J. Pratt (1974, p. 106) comments that "a frequently overlooked, but quite significant factor in this development has been the increased organized activity on the part of senior citizens themselves." Though not allied with a political party, these organizations are working toward fairly definite positions on the issues mentioned below. The largest of these organizations, the American Association of Retired Persons, has grown in membership from 2 million in 1969 to 8.8 million in 1975. Norval D. Glenn (1974), writing on "Aging and Conservatism," suggests that the attitudes and values of people tend to stabilize and become resistant to change as they grow through middle age. But, he concludes, "although the evidence suggests that attitudes probably become somewhat less susceptible to change as people grow older, there is scant evidence for any other contribution of aging to conservatism" (p. 176).

As issues arise that affect the economic welfare of the elderly, it seems likely that the older voters will make their wishes known in local congressional elections and local state elections, and that political candidates will be aware of this. Thus the elderly voters may make their influence felt on issues that are essentially nonpartisan. The issues will probably center around:

1. Social Security legislation
2. Age discrimination in employment
3. Housing for the elderly
4. Social Services for the elderly
5. National Health Insurance

The national organizations of older people will take definite positions on these issues and will attempt to organize the elderly voters for political action. These national organizations may not attempt to form a single coalition for political action. No doubt they will differ somewhat among themselves on specific issues. But they will almost certainly be together in a broad way, and this will be clearly visible to the members of the Congress, as well as to members of state legislatures.

Educational Status and Interests of the Elderly. As the 20th century draws to a close, the educational activity of adults, and especially of older people, will increase. The level of formal schooling is more closely related to participation in adult education than any other socioeconomic factor. If present trends continue, that level will increase dramatically. According to census data the median number of school years completed by those 65 and over in the U.S.A. in 1950 was 8.1. In 1970 the median had risen to only 8.7, but it is estimated that by 1990 the median will have jumped to 11.9 or just short of a high school education.

At present there are many older people who feel that they are too old to learn or that they do not have enough time to devote to further education. Houle (1975) cites a contemporary study made by the Educational Testing Service of a national sample of people aged 55–60. Many of these people said they would like to engage in continuing education but felt they could not succeed at it. These people were then asked what kept them from studying what they wanted to learn. The chief reasons given by people aged 55–60 were: too old, 42 percent; not enough time, 40 percent; cost, 36 percent; do not want full-time schooling, 34 percent; job responsibilities, 23 percent; home responsibilities, 22 percent; time requirement for the program, 19 percent; not enough energy, 15 percent; and attendance requirements, 15 percent. It seems likely that a mind-set against formal education has been established in this group. But since the coming generation of the elderly will have a median formal educational level of high school graduation, this mind-set will probably be weakened.

Houle (1975) has made a very positive case for the values of continuing education to older people, summarizing his views as follows:

In the past, education for the elderly has been viewed as an activity which, like needlework or croquet, was a pleasant but non-essential way of filling some of the abundant leisure time of the aged. As a contrast, I suggest that education throughout adulthood but particularly education for the young-old and the old-old can yield specific and highly important returns to the individual and to society. Episodes of learning, with their individual challenges and accomplishments, might well offer to old people the task orientation which is so often missing from much of their activity. After years of striving to accomplish specific deeds and overcome specific challenges, old people often find retirement to be generally void of meaningful activities. Perhaps if education is properly addressed to the interests and needs of the elderly, particularly those whose minds have been kept alert by constant use, it can offer challenges which many people feel to be missing. Whether or not this result is possible has yet to be proved but it raises a basic, unanswered question which must be addressed if there is to be any meaningful understanding of education for old people (p. 15).

Continuing education, or study programs taken formally or informally during adult years, has grown a great deal in the United States since 1950. Regularly scheduled study groups, discussion groups, and lecture series may be sponsored by universities, churches, labor unions, employers, public school systems, libraries, and community centers. Counting all such groups, Johnstone and Rivera (1965) found that in 1961–1962, in a national sample of adults who were not engaged in regular university study, the age distribution of those in some form of continuing education was 22 percent for those aged 40–49, 13 percent for those 50–59, 6 percent for those 60–69, and 2 percent for those over 70. A study made by the Educational Testing Service (Houle, 1974) in 1972 found that 31 percent of persons aged 18–60 who were not full-time students had engaged in some form of continuing education during the year.

It has been noted that participation in continuing education is closely related to the level of formal education achieved by a person. That is, university graduates are much more likely to take part in continuing education than are persons who have not graduated from high school. A study of a representative sample of out-of-school American adults aged 18–60 showed that the extent of participation in continuing education rose steadily with each increment of formal schooling. Only 10 percent of those who had one to eight years of instruction took some part in some kind of adult education, while 57 percent of those who had had at least a college education were engaged in such activity (Carp, Peterson, & Roelfs, 1974).

EFFECTS OF AN INCREASED EDUCATIONAL LEVEL. It is being tacitly or explicitly assumed that the increasing educational level of the elderly population will give them greater competence and also will lead them to want more continuing education. This sounds reasonable to a group of educators, but if it proves to be true, many of the future students in programs of continuing education will be people of the lower white-collar class and the upper working class and thus will differ in social class from present-day students in adult classes. This raises the question whether the 20 percent of elders who will be college graduates at the end of the century will display the behavior and attitudes of the seven percent who are college graduates today.

The Harris Poll opens up some interesting questions in this connection. This writer (Havighurst, 1976) has studied the results of the Harris Poll in relation to the educational level of the respondents. Respondents who are college graduates were compared with respondents with less education. In general, the group with a college education is more active, more achievement oriented, shows greater life satisfaction, and acknowledges fewer personal problems when compared with the group with less education. They do more reading and studying; they participate more in political and civic activities; they do more unpaid volunteer work. In general, they seem to act "younger" than those with less education.

It will be important to monitor the activities and interests of the college graduates of the future to find out what kind of interests they have in continuing education, and how they make use of their greater amount of education as senior citizens and workers.

THE INTERMEDIATE FUTURE—1990–2030

We have noted that the near future, 1978–1990, which can be projected from the contemporary situation, is likely to be a rather stable period for the elderly, except for the uncertainty caused by monetary inflation. But the intermediate future, 1990–2030, may usher in drastic changes in the situation of the elderly, which cannot be foretold with much assurance.

It is now pretty generally agreed by the experts on the economics and the technology of the United States that the gross national product will undergo a reduced rate of per capita growth, but that there will continue to be some growth. This will be related, in important ways, to the increased cost of energy. In 1975 the Energy Center at the University of Florida reported that the amount of energy that could be bought in the form of gasoline for $1 in 1965 cost $2 in 1965 dollars, and even more in 1975 dollars. The 20th century industrialization of the "affluent third" of the world's people has been based essentially on cheap petroleum, steel, aluminum, lumber, paper, plastics, and fertilizers. These are now increasingly scarce and expensive. By the year 2000 the world's supply of petroleum and natural gas will be nearly used up, if the present rate of use continues. Coal will be available for at least a century but will cost more in human labor per unit of energy than petroleum has cost.

These trends will cause major changes in the material standard of living and in life-styles, especially, at first, of young and middle-aged adults. By 1990 they will probably affect the lives of elderly people as well, and in ways that will interrupt the stability which we have projected for the coming decade.

After 1990, employment, income, and life-styles of any adult age group will depend upon the following factors:

- The gross national product per capita, the distribution of this product among the various groups of people, and its distribution in terms of consumption versus capital investment.
- The demand of the economy for human labor.
- The cost of energy.
- The distribution of the working population between the sexes and among various age groups.

To look ahead into the intermediate future, we need data on these matters, or at least estimates based upon our best judgments. The probable age distribution in the United States is presented in Table 1.1, with special attention to the sizes and relative proportions of the age groups 20–64 and 65–74. The sizes of these two age groups are important because, although nearly all the work of the nation will be done by people aged 20–74, the subgroup 65–74 will probably be seen as marginal, a group with less moral claim to employment and less working capacity than the 20–64 group. Furthermore, the constructive induction of the 15–24 age group into the labor force is a critical need for the health of the society, and may be given priority over employment of the 65–74 group.

Two age groups are essentially "marginal" to the labor force —the 65–74 group and the 15–24 group. The older group can be encouraged to leave the labor force by increased retirement payments. The younger group cannot be held out of the labor force without real moral concern by the society as a whole. They do not have an acceptable alternative to employment, except for those who want and need more formal education. And the 1975–1985 period is critical for the 15–24 age group because they will number 40 million in the 1975–1980 period and 35 million in the 1985–1990 period, because of the high birth rates between 1954 and 1961. The birth rate dropped by about 25 percent between 1961 and 1971. Thus, after 1990, the proportion of the population that is 15–24 years old will be substantially lower than the equivalent proportion in 1975–1985.

The Future Cost of Energy. The cost of energy during the first half of the 21st century is a matter which will depend not only upon research but also upon political action during the remainder of the present century. In 1975 the United States consumed about 30 percent of the energy used in the entire world, for its six percent of the world's population. Basically, the cost of energy will control the socioeconomic structure of the 21st century. It will determine the numbers and age structure of the labor force. It will affect the distribution of the population between big cities and smaller cities. It will affect the structure and size of dwelling units. In short, it will have a substantial impact on the life-styles, incomes, and activities of the elderly.

Alternatives for the Life of the Elderly After 1990. The most generally accepted prediction for the United States and the Western European countries is that the cost of a unit of energy in the year 2000 will be at least four times what it was in 1970. At the same time the most generally accepted prediction on population is that those countries will achieve a zero population growth between 2000 and 2050, with the United States reaching zero growth by about 2050. This is the assumption on which the population projections of Table 1 are based.

If these assumptions prove true, how will the life-styles and values of elderly people respond?

ALTERNATIVE ENERGY POLICIES. If we assume the continuation of a democratic political structure probably moving toward somewhat greater government participation in the economy, and if we assume that there will be no major war, we may describe two contrasting energy futures, both tolerable for a population which has achieved zero population growth and which has come to terms with the need to maintain an equilibrium between the use of energy and critical materials and the creation and restoration of the same.

The proper utilization of human resources and the education and development of human beings will be essential for both alternatives. The success of the society will depend on the efficiency with which energy, capital, and labor are used.

The alternative energy futures have been described recently in a major paper by Amory B. Lovins (1976), a British physicist. Lovins describes two very different policies and programs for meeting the world's energy needs over the next 50 years:

A. *Obtaining Energy from Continuing Replaceable Sources.* This means energy from the sun, which consists of direct solar radiation, wind, tides, hydroelectric power, ocean thermal gradients, and which, through photosynthesis, produces the annual plant growth on the earth, called bio-mass. Major attention will be given to more efficient use of energy in the U.S.A.

B. *Obtaining Energy from Nonreplaceable Sources.* This refers to energy from fossil fuels, including coal, petroleum, and natural gas; or from atomic energy, including atomic fission or nuclear fusion. Though the transformation of matter into energy in nuclear reactors does use up a certain amount of matter, the actual mass of matter turned into energy is small and does not threaten the existence of the earth. But there are other dangers to human life and human society which must be considered.

At present the more or less official American policy is B—using fossil fuels, especially coal, increasingly for a couple of decades, while enormously expanding the atomic power industry at a very high cost in capital investment. By the year 2025, petroleum and natural gas would be practially all used up, and more than half the energy needs of the U.S.A. would be met by nuclear power plants. There would be a major problem of safe storage of poisonous radioactive waste materials which will be dangerous for thousands of years, and nuclear energy technology would be shared with many other countries, all of which would obtain the means of waging nuclear warfare.

However there is growing public pressure for alternative A— turning to energy from continuing replaceable sources, mainly the sun. This policy would be tied to a program of more efficient use of energy in the United States, which now uses its energy resources only two-thirds as efficiently as do the western European nations, with their more efficient passenger and freight transportation systems. Lovins cites energy use research studies which show that the U.S.A. can double the efficiency of use of energy by the year 2000, and by 2040 can reduce the per capita use or consumption of primary energy to one-third of today's performance. This would require no reduction of physical comfort by Americans, but they would use more efficient automobile engines, more bus service, more railroad passenger service, and more efficient heating methods for homes and commercial buildings. By 2025, the U.S.A. would be almost exclusively using energy from replaceable sources—the sun. And the U.S.A. would be using less energy than it is today, though it would have a population approaching 300 million.

The significance of the two alternative energy futures is indicated in Table 1.7.

Effects on the Elderly Population. The two futures will differ most, from the point of view of the elderly, in the use the society makes of them as workers, and in the access they have to jobs and earned income. Alternative A will cause more employment of workers, with minimized expenditure of mechanical energy. Alternative B will present an energy-intensive technology, with much capital invested in labor-saving machinery. Both alternatives will produce enough goods and services to raise the material standard of living above the present average level; but alternative B will give people more leisure than alternative A. It appears likely that alternative A will produce a high degree of ego involvement and of work satisfaction on the part of workers, with more attention to skillful use of tools and on easy human relations at the work place. Alternative B will use more mass production and assembly-line methods and will generate a somewhat higher average per capita income than will alternative A.

MATERIAL STANDARD OF LIVING.   A major increase of costs of energy and certain scarce critical materials will tend to lower the material standard of living. People will probably respond by working more years or longer hours to increase the production of goods and services, and thus to maintain the present standard of living. Therefore it appears likely that elderly people will be encouraged to stay in the labor force as long as they are reasonably productive. One may even imagine that the notion of mandatory retirement at a fixed age will be forgotten, and the average age of retirement may go up to about 70. There may be a considerable development of part-time employment.

This trend would suggest that there will be more emphasis on research with the aim of fitting work assignments to persons with the skills and strength appropriate to these jobs. The work of Koyl (1969) in matching persons and jobs after the age of 50 is likely to be developed, as well as that of Belbin (1972) in retraining older workers for new jobs.

PERSONAL INCOME: EARNINGS AND RETIREMENT INCOME. With a longer working life and therefore a shorter retirement, the

Social Security program and private pension programs will be substantially modified, necessitating lower Social Security taxes and smaller pension trust funds. The goal of a 60 to 70 percent replacement income after retirement will be easier to achieve, because the average duration of the period of retirement will be decreased by five to ten years.

HOUSING. The living quarters of people need energy for heat, air conditioning, lighting, and cooking. The cost of these facilities will rise, possibly enough to cause home builders to seek greater efficiency in the supply and use of energy. The net effect may be that each person will inhabit fewer square feet of living space. This will apply to all age groups, but especially to elderly couples and singles, whose space needs are not great. It is likely that multiple-unit housing will be designed for the economic use of energy, and also for the collection and use of solar energy. Similar action will probably take place in the construction of subsidized public housing for low-income elderly.

RESIDENTIAL ARRANGEMENTS FOR THE ELDERLY. An interesting and possibly important response to the rising costs of energy and food (farming uses 14 percent of the energy consumed in this country) may be the creation of colonies of middle-class and upper working class elderly couples on the outskirts of big cities, with gardens, orchards, and small dairies. People aged 60 to 75 may be interested in living in such areas, where they might produce up to half of the food they need through a kind of producer-consumer cooperative. They could freeze vegetables and store fruit and root vegetables for year-round use. Some could keep a few milk cows, and some might like to produce butter and cheese for their own consumption. Working two to four hours a day would keep them happily occupied. Bus service to the commercial and theater centers and to libraries and churches would keep them in touch with younger family members and old friends.

Less interesting but equally necessary will be a systematic program designed to help older people who are living alone in the inner city, in small apartments and single rooms in low-cost residential hotels. Studies of the elderly in big cities (Bild and Ha-

Table 1.7 Impact of Two Alternative Energy Sources

Impact	A. Energy from continuing replaceable sources	B. Energy from non-replaceable sources
Use of human labor	High. More jobs. More labor-intensive technology	Medium. Greater man-hour productivity
Use of capital	High initially, for new energy-collecting and converting industries	Very high, due to high capital cost of nuclear energy plants
Efficiency of use of energy	High	Medium
Quality of product	High	High

Ego-involvement of workers	High	Medium
Material standard of living	Medium-high	High, if new nuclear energy technology is successful
Pollution of environ- ment	Low	High. Might become a major danger to human life.

vighurst, 1976) show that this group is severely disadvantaged because of poor health, loneliness, and alienation. Senior centers and church organizations attempt to serve these people today, and presumably will be the major resources in the intermediate future. There seems to be no quick and easy solution to this problem.

CIVIC-POLITICAL ACTION. We noted earlier that there is no national political movement of the elderly, and neither political party appears to have the allegiance of a majority of older voters. However older people exert influence on legislatures and Congress in connection with specific government actions, such as linking Social Security benefits to the purchasing power of the dollar, and providing federal and state government support for state and local programs for the elderly.

It seems probable that this kind of united action by older people will become more evident and more decisive as the cost of energy rises and as human labor is more in demand. For example, after 1980, when the current crisis of unemployed youth has somewhat abated as a result of decreasing numbers in the 15–25 age group, it is probable that through such organizations as the American Association of Retired Persons, the National Council of Senior Citizens, and the Grey Panthers, senior citizens will push to amend the Age Discrimination in Employment Act so as to raise the age level covered by the Act up to 70 from the present 65. Thus the economic position of the elderly will become more and more a conscious concern of older people in their political and educational activity.

CONCLUSION

If we accept the proposition that the development and use of energy resources will dominate the civic-political arena by the year 2000, and since the situation in the year 2000 depends so much on research and development yet to come, it seems wise to set up a task force on planning for the elderly that will monitor technological developments and socioeconomic developments during the next 15 years. Then, by about 1990, the task force might come forward with a statement of the issues that bear upon the needs of the elderly population and present a program for social and civic action.

REFERENCES

Belbin, R. M., & Belbin, E. *Problems in adult retraining.* London: Heinemann, 1972.

Bild, B., & Havighurst, R. J. Senior citizens in great cities: The case of Chicago. *Gerontologist,* 1976, *16,* (1, Part 2).

Binstock, R. Aging and the future of American politics. *The Annals,* 1974, *415,* 176–186.

Carp, A., Peterson, R., & Roelfs, P. Adult learning interests and experiences. In P. Cross & J. R. Valley, (Eds.), *Planning for non-traditional programs.* San Francisco: Jossey-Bass, 1974.

Glenn, N. Aging and conservatism. *The Annals,* 1974, *415,* 176–186.

Golant, S. Residential concentrations of the future elderly. *Gerontologist,* 1975, *15* (1, Part 2), 16–23.

Havighurst, R. J. *Aging in America: Implications for education.* Washington, D.C.: National Council on the Aging, 1976.

Havighurst, R. J., & deVries, A. Life styles and free time activities of retired men. *Human Development,* 1969, *12,* 34–54.

Houle, C. O. *Continuing education for the elderly.* Unpublished research paper. Committee on Human Development, The University of Chicago, 1975.

Johnstone, J. W. C., & Rivera, R. J. *Volunteers for learning.* Chicago: Aldine, 1965.

Koyl, L. F., & Hansen, P. M. *Age, physical ability, and work potential.* Washington, D.C.: National Council on the Aging, 1969.

Koyl, L., & Youry, M. Gulhemp: What workers can do. *Manpower,* 1975, *7*(6), 4–9.

Lovins, A. B. Energy strategy: The road not taken? *Foreign Affairs,* 1976, *55,* 65–96.

National Council on the Aging. *The myth and reality of aging.* Washington, D.C.: National Council on the Aging, 1975.

Parnes, H. S., et al. *The pre-retirement years: Five years in the work lives of middle-aged men.* Columbus, Ohio: Center for Human Resources Research, Ohio State University, 1974.

Pratt, H. J. Old age associations in national politics. *The Annals,* 1974, *415,* 176–186.

U.S. Department of Commerce, Bureau of the Census. *Current Population Reports*, Series P-25, No. 601. Washington, D.C.: U.S. Government Printing Office, 1975.

U.S. Department of Commerce, Bureau of the Census. *Current Population Reports*, Series P-23, No. 59. Washington, D.C.: U.S. Government Printing Office, 1976.

U.S. Department of Labor, Bureau of Labor Statistics. *Employment and unemployment in 1974*. Special Labor Force Report 178. Washington, D.C.: U.S. Government Printing Office, 1975.

U.S. Senate Special Committee on Aging. *Hearing before the Subcommittee on Employment and Retirement Incomes*. Statement by Marshall M. Holbeb, Chairman, Illinois State Council on Aging. Chicago: August 14, 1975.

-2-
Changing Demography and Dependency Costs: The Implications of Future Dependency Ratios and Their Composition

Robert L. Clark and Joseph J. Spengler

In all societies individuals who are engaged in productive activities must produce enough to support themselves and that proportion of the population that is currently not contributing to the nation's output of goods and services. These nonproductive members of society include those who have not yet entered the labor force, those who have retired from the labor force, and those who are of working age but are not employed either by choice or by economic circumstance. This chapter examines the present and future costs of publicly financed support programs for the young and the old. Although we allow labor force participation rates of the working age population to vary, the dependent population in our model refers, except as otherwise noted, to the number of individuals 0–18 and 65 years and over.

In 1974, 33.8 percent of the U.S. population were young dependents and another 10.3 percent were 65 and older. Federal government expenditures financing education, health care, and income security programs plus spending by state and local governments on educational programs that directly benefited the dependent populations totaled $140 billion, or 14.2 percent of disposable personal income (DPI). This research will examine the future trend of these dependency costs, with the assumption that fertility rates will remain near the replacement level.

To be able to estimate the proportion of national income required to support dependents, the future age structure of the population must be calculated. In the following section, projections of the Bureau of the Census are used to derive the age structure for various years between 1974 and 2050. The subsequent three sections analyze the interrelation between the population age structure and the ability of the work force to support a changing dependent population. The relative cost of public support for young and old dependents is estimated in the penultimate section. Because the elderly require more public expenditure per dependent, the total proportion of DPI needed to finance all dependents is expected, within the framework of our model, to rise from 14.2 percent to 16.2 percent in 2050. Finally, we explore additional factors which may influence the future dependency burden.

POPULATION GROWTH

If current low fertility rates are maintained, one of the most pressing economic issues facing the nation could be, but need not be, the changing age structure and its impact on the size and composition of the dependent population. In addition to fertility, mortality and net immigration influence the age structure and size of the population. New population projections reflect errors in past expectations concerning fertility and mortality, and the inference that these expectations need to be adjusted. The future size and age composition of the population will depend mainly upon the course of fertility. Fluctuations in the annual number of births can introduce irregularities into the age structure which, 20 or so years later, introduce fluctuations in the population approximately 20 years of age, and hence in the number of births to women in their early 20s.

Population growth in the future depends upon the course of mortality and net immigration together with the behavior of total fertility. A further decrease in mortality will not add greatly to population growth. Given the 1973 age-specific mortality rates, 67 percent of white males and 82 percent of white females reached age 65. Were the main causes of death reduced by one-fourth, male life expectancy at age 65 would be raised from 13.13 years to 15.82, and female life expectancy at age 65 from 17.15 years to 19.93. Corresponding increases at age 45 would be from 27.47 to 30.92 for men, and from 33.50 to 36.85 for women. However, "it would require a major breakthrough in research to effect a reduction of as much as one-fourth in the number of deaths from any one cause" (Metropolitan Life Insurance Company, 1975). Accordingly, although some life extension is still to be expected, it will not significantly modify age structure. Indeed, life extension exercises little influence upon the relative number of older persons in a population unless life expectancy at, for example, 70 is decidedly higher than now. Thus, given an unlikely life expectancy at birth of 90 years, slightly over 30 percent of a stationary population would be over age 59, compared with about 21 percent if the life expectancy were 70 (United Nations, 1956).

Since net legal immigration has been running in the neighborhood of 400,000 per year, the projections of the Bureau of the Census, including immigration, rest upon the assumption of an annual net immigration of 400,000. As we indicate below, this inflow contributes to population growth unless it tends to depress fertility (Coale, 1972). The actual volume of net immigration has been in excess of 400,000, since many persons enter the country illegally. For example, in the 12 months ending in June 1975, the Immigration Service turned back 800,000 foreigners who attempted to enter the United States improperly and arrested 757,000 who succeeded in getting past the border (Fogel, 1975).

Given the limited contribution of mortality reduction and immigration, population growth in the future will depend almost entirely on the behavior of fertility. Therefore errors in popula-

tion projections are most likely to originate in erroneous estimates of future fertility and not in underestimation of net
immigration or mortality. It now appears that total fertility will
settle in the neighborhood of the replacement level, or 2.1.
Should this supposition be borne out, total population, together
with its age structure, will develop as summarized in Tables 2.1
and 2.2. Of course, even given replacement-level fertility, the
timing of births as reflected in the mean age of childbearing will
modify population size. For example, we use the Bureau of Census projection Series II based on an ultimate mean age of childbearing of 26 years, together with an annual net immigration of
400,000. This series is summarized in Table 2.3 along with Series
II-X, which corresponds to II, but with net immigration put at
zero. We do not include a Series II-L, which assumes a mean age
of childbearing of 28 years. With the population at 212 million
in 1974, these series, together with Series II-R which allows fertility to vary with cohort size, develop as indicated in Table 2.4.

Whereas late timing of births slows growth somewhat (cf. II
and II-L), elimination of net immigration produces a 48 million
population difference by 2050 (cf. II and II-X); this figure is too
low because clandestine immigration raises the total volume of
net immigration above 400,000 per year. Of course, with total
fertility at 1.7 instead of 2.1 as in Series III, even with net immigration continuing at 400,000 per year, population levels off at
251.8 million in 2015–2020 and then begins to decline, falling to
226.7 million by 2050 (Table 2.3).

POPULATION COMPOSITION

Table 2.1 presents a projection to the year 2050 based on the
assumptions that net annual immigration is 400,000 per year, the
mean childbearing age is 26, there is a slight increase in life
expectancy and that total fertility is at 2.1, the replacement level.
Table 2.2, based on the same assumptions, presents significant
age-based ratios and fractions for the purposes of this chapter.
Table 2.3 contrasts the ratios in Tables 2.1 and 2.2—both based
on the assumption of total fertility at the replacement level and

net immigration at 400,000 per year—with Projection Series II-X, which is similar to Series II except for the assumption that net immigration is zero. Series III is based on the assumption that total fertility is below the replacement level while annual net immigration remains at 400,000.

Reading across Table 2.2 from left to right indicates the following movements:

1. The fraction of the population in the 0–17 age bracket decreases to a near stable level.
2. The fraction above age 54 increases.
3. The fractions in age categories lying between age 18 and ages 54–64 increase, but then decline slightly below their peaks.
4. The fraction in age group 18–69 moves up to something like a plateau.
5. The ratio of those in age categories 18 to 54–69 to those in higher age categories declines.

Comparison of Series II with Series II-X does not reveal much difference between the fraction in the 18–64 group and those 65 and over. Turning to Series III, however, we find that the ratio of those 18–64 to those 65 and over is significantly lower because of an increase in the fraction over 65 as a result of the lowness of fertility.

AGE STRUCTURE AND LABOR FORCE

The dependency ratio of a population is conditioned principally by when individuals enter the labor force and when they withdraw from it, as well as by the age structure of the population. Participation in the labor force by males is lower today than in the past, in part because years in educational institutions have increased and because many who enter the labor force leave it earlier than was customary in the past. Male labor force participation has declined significantly among those under 15 and over 54 since the late 1940s and early 1950s, resulting in a lower market activity rate for all males 16 and over. Overall labor force participation is slightly higher, however, than it was in the late 1940s

Table 2.1 Projected Age Structure, 1975-2050 (Millions)[a]

Age group	1975	1990	2000	2025	2050
Total	213.5	245.1	262.5	299.7	318.4
0-14	53.8	70.5	58.6	62.1	65.5
15-17	12.5	9.7	12.5	12.8	13.2
0-17	66.3	67.7	71.1	74.9	78.7
18-54	105.1	128.0	137.9	142.3	152.3
35 and over	42.1	49.4	53.5	82.2	87.4
62 and over	27.7	35.0	36.4	58.7	61.9
18-61	112.2	132.4	155.0	165.8	177.8

18-64	124.9	148.5	160.8	176.4	188.5
65 and over	22.3	28.9	30.6	48.1	51.2
18-69	133.0	158.4	171.8	(192.6)[b]	(205.2)
70 and over	14.2	19.0	21.6	(31.9)	(34.5)
18 and over	147.2	177.4	191.4	224.5	239.7
Median age	28.8	32.3	34.8	36.9	37.0

[a] Assuming total fertility rate of 2.1, a net annual immigration of 400,000, a mean childbearing age of 26, and a slight increase in life expectancy.
[b] Figures in brackets are our estimates.
Source: U.S. Bureau of the Census (1975).

Table 2.2 Projected Age Structure, 1975–2050 (Fractions)[a]

Age group	1975	1990	2000	2025	2050
Total (millions)	213.5	245.1	262.5	299.7	318.4
Total (fraction)	1.00	1.00	1.00	1.00	1.00
0-17	0.31	0.28	0.27	0.25	0.25
55 and over	0.20	0.20	0.20	0.27	0.27
62 and over	0.13	0.14	0.14	0.20	0.19
65 and over	0.10	0.12	0.12	0.16	0.16
69 and over	0.07	0.07	0.08	0.11	0.11
18-54	0.49	0.52	0.53	0.47	0.48

18-61	0.53	0.54	0.59	0.55	0.56
18-64	0.59	0.61	0.61	0.59	0.59
18-69	0.62	0.65	0.65	0.64	0.64
18-54/55+	2.5	2.6	2.6	1.7	1.7
18-61/62+	4.1	3.8	4.2	2.8	2.9
18-64/65+	5.6	5.1	5.3	3.7	3.7
18-69/70+	9.3	8.3	8.0	6.0	5.9
Median age	28.8	32.3	34.8	36.9	37.0

aSame assumptions as Table 1.
Source: U.S. Bureau of the Census (1975).

Table 2.3 Population Projections, 1975–2050

Age group	1974–75	1990	2000	2025	2050
Series II[a]					
0–17	67.3	67.7	71.1	74.8	78.7
18–64	122.8	148.5	160.8	176.8	188.5
65 and over	21.8	28.9	30.6	48.1	51.2
Total	211.9	245.1	262.5	299.7	318.4
18–64/total	0.58	0.61	0.61	0.59	0.59
18–64/65+	5.7	5.1	5.25	3.7	3.7
Median age	28.8	32.3	34.8	36.9	37.0
Series II–x[b]					
0–17	67.3	64.8	66.5	65.9	65.6
18–64	122.8	143.8	152.4	154.7	158.6
65 and over	21.8	28.8	30.2	45.7	45.8
Total	211.9	237.4	249.1	269.3	270.0
18–64/total	0.58	0.61	0.61	0.57	0.59
18–64/65+	5.7	5.0	5.0	3.38	3.46
Median age	28.8	32.6	35.4	37.7	37.8

Series III[c]

0-17	67.3	.58.2	57.3	49.9	44.1
18-64	122.8	148.5	157.2	152.4	135.6
65 and over	21.8	28.9	30.6	48.1	47.0
Total	211.9	235.6	245.1	250.4	226.7
18-64/total	0.58	0.63	0.64	0.61	0.6
18-64/65+	5.7	5.1	5.1	3.17	2.89
Median age	28.8	33.4	37.0	41.8	42.6

[a] Assumptions same as Table 2.
[b] Assumptions same as Table 2, but net immigration assumed to be 0, not 400,000.
[c] Same assumptions as Table 2, but fertility assumed to be 1.7, not 2.1.
Source: U.S. Bureau of the Census (1975).

Table 2.4 Bureau of Census Population Projections (Millions)

Year	II	II-L	II-R	II-X
1980	222.8	221.8	222.0	220.2
2000	262.5	255.5	259.5	249.1
2025	299.7	285.9	294.5	269.3
2050	318.4	299.1	305.3	270.0

Source: U.S. Bureau of the Census (1975).

because total female labor force participation has increased enough to offset slight decreases in total male labor force participation (U.S. Department of Labor, 1975). Moreover, projections of male and female labor force participation (Johnston, 1973) suggest that while labor force participation is expected to be lower among males by 1990, female labor force participation is expected to increase enough to elevate overall participation slightly above the 1970 level. The interrelation between fertility and the participation of women in market activity is reflected both in the fact that being employed adversely affects fertility and that the household responsibility of child rearing is a leading cause of the withdrawal of women from the labor force.

We may say that the *potential capacity* of a population to produce output and to maintain a high worker-dependent ratio is at or near a peak when a population is stationary (all other things being equal). For example, if fertility is at the replacement level, the percentage of males of working age, say 18–64, in the resulting stationary population is about 60 percent, or about two percent higher than if this population were growing at 0.5 percent per year (Coale & Demeny, 1966). With something like 60 percent of the population of working age and in the labor force, the ratio of the labor force to those outside it and dependent on it is 1.5:1. If, however, five units of these 60 transfer to the dependent category and augment it to 45, the worker-dependent ratio declines to $(60 - 5)/(40 + 5)$, or 1.22:1. And if 10 transfer, the ratio falls to 50/50 or 1:1, one-third below the original 1.5:1. Thus, with fertility at the replacement level, the average age of retirement is a decisive factor influencing the productive potential of the economy.

THE DEPENDENCY RATIO AND THE EFFECTS OF RETIREMENT AGE ON THE RATIO

Dependency ratios can be expressed either as the ratio of workers to dependents (as in the previous section) or as the ratio of dependents to workers. Using the latter definition, Table 2.5 lists the dependency ratios through 2050.

Table 2.5 Projected Dependency Ratios, 1975–2050[a] (Percentages)

Year	Age 0-17	65 and over	Total
1975	53.1	17.9	71
1990	45.6	19.5	65.1
2000	44.2	19.0	63.2
2025	42.5	27.3	69.8
2050	41.8	27.2	69

[a] Same assumptions as Table 2.

While it is sometimes suggested that the burden on the work-ing-age population will not be much affected by the aging of the population, since old dependents merely replace young depen-dents, this inference is not likely to be true over the next 75 years. It is much more likely that this burden will increase somewhat, as argued in the next section.

Future costs of supporting old-age-connected and youth-con-nected government programs depend on several factors:

1. The numerator and denominator which comprise the ratio. (Are more dependents being supported by fewer workers?)
2. The composition of the ratio. (What proportion of the dependents are old and what proportion young?)
3. The per-person costs of government support of young dependents compared to outlays on older dependents.

As Table 5 indicates, the dependency ratio is likely to remain relatively stable, and may even decline a bit. However the propor-tion of old to young will increase. Moreover, the total govern-ment outlay for each older dependent is likely to be higher than the outlay for each young dependent. (We present data to illustrate this point in the next section.) In addition, the proportion of older dependents may increase even further if the strong movement toward early retirement continues.

An increase in the tax burden on people of working age is made even more likely by the existence of a strong movement toward early retirement. If this continues, the fraction of the population of working age may decline somewhat further, since older dependents will include not only those 65 and over, but a growing fraction of those under 65. In other words, it is not only the aging of the population as such that can elevate the overall dependency ratio, but also a decline in labor force participation on the part of those in the 55–64 age group.

The next several paragraphs will illustrate the impact of early retirement. For those readers who may not wish to follow the symbols, they illustrate the following basic point:

With taxes to finance dependency costs and average earnings given, the average benefit paid to retirees depends upon the ratio of employed workers to retirees. The fewer the workers per retiree, the lower the benefit level per retiree. Alternatively, rising tax rates would be needed to finance a constant relative benefit to the elderly as the worker/retiree ratio declines.

To illustrate the impact of early retirement, we can proceed as follows: Let L denote the labor force; e, the fraction of it employed; R, the retirees; y, the average earnings of employed workers that are subject to a tax to finance dependency costs; i, the average benefit of retirees; t, the tax imposed on y, all of which is subject to the tax; and r, the ratio of i to y. Then,

$$i = (t \cdot y \cdot L \cdot e)/R$$

$$r = i/y = (t \cdot L \cdot e)/R$$

Thus, the magnitude of i varies directly with t, L, y, and e, and inversely with R; whereas r varies directly with t, L, and e, and inversely with R. Of primary concern here, however, is the fact that, with t and y given, i depends upon $(e \cdot L/R)$, that is, upon the ratio of *employed* workers to retirees. It is true, of course, that t not only can be increased, but can be made incident on a larger fraction of earnings y, if not all is subject to taxation as we assume above. But this extension is deemed burdensome as is an increase in the taxed fraction of y.

If we set $e = 1$ and $t = 0.1$, then $r = 0.1(L/R)$. The value of r ranges from 0.1 to 0.4 accordingly as L/R varies between 1 and 4. If the tax is higher than 0.1, the value of r is proportionately higher as follows:

L/R	$t = 0.1$	$t = 0.2$
4	$r = 0.4$	$r = 0.8$
3	$r = 0.3$	$r = 0.6$
2	$r = 0.2$	$r = 0.4$
1	$r = 0.1$	$r = 0.2$

Let us now turn to how the value of L/R will vary in the year 2050 with the age of retirement at which, by assumption, everyone withdraws from the labor force L and enters the retirement category R. The following calculations are made by using the proportion of the population that will be in each age category in 2050.

1. (18–64)/(65 and over) = 60.09/15.95 = 3.77 = L/R.
2. (18–59)/(60 and over) = 54.37/21.67 = 2.51 = L/R.
3. (18–54)/(55 and over) = 48.28/27.76 = 1.74 = L/R.

Should everyone remain in the labor force through age 69, the value of L/R would approximate 6. Thus

4. (18–69)/(70 and over) = 65.24/10.80 = 6.04 = L/R.

These figures are based on a stable male stationary population as described by Coale and Demeny (1966).

The economic tolerability of a worker-dependent ratio turns ultimately upon productivity per worker and the average material level of living desired by a population. Suppose that net national product per employed member of the labor force, w, is 100, that half the population P needs to be employed and half dependent, and that average consumption, $c = 50$, satisfies the population.

Then, with $w = 2c$, and $0.5\ Pw = Pc$, only half of P needs to be employed. If, however, we raise desired average consumption by 50 percent but are unable to increase w, we must increase the fraction of P in the labor force to 0.75, since then $0.75\ Pw = 1.5\ Pc$. In short, how low the ratio of the labor force to the population can be reduced, together with the ratio of the labor force to those not in the labor force, depends upon the ratio of *desired average consumption* to *average output* per member of the labor force.

CURRENT AND FUTURE DEPENDENCY COSTS

In this section we estimate the influence of low fertility rates on the support levels needed to finance social programs for young and old dependents. Table 2.6 shows the expenditures in 1974 by the federal government on health, education, and income maintenance programs according to the age group of beneficiaries

Table 2.6   Federal Expenditures (Billions of Dollars) in 1974 for Programs Whose Benefits Accrue Directly to Youths and the Elderly Plus State and Local Expenditures for Educational Programs

Item	Youths 0-18	Elderly 65 & older
Education[a]	59.8	—
Child care[b]	.4	—
Health care[b]	2.2	13.5
Income security[c]	10.5	53.5
Total	72.9	67.0

[a] Allocates all expenditures on elementary and secondary schools to youth expenditures. Also includes college expenditures for 18-year-olds.

[b] Includes federal expenditures on Medicare, Medicaid and other health outlays that can be allocated by age of beneficiary; does not include state or local contributions.

[c] The federally funded income security programs are: Social Security; pension expenditures for railroad employees, federal civilian employees, uniformed service members and coal miners' widows; public assistance; income-tested veterans' pensions; AFDC; and in-kind assistance other than health care.

Source: National Center for Education Statistics (1975); Office of Management and Budget (1975); Council of Economic Advisers (1976).

combined with state and local expenditures on educational programs. These figures indicate that the estimated public expenditure on youths was $72.9 billion, while benefits totaling $67
billion were paid to those aged 65 and over. Thus dependency
costs were approximately $140 billion or 14.2 percent of DPI.
Obviously these expenditures do not reflect all of the publicly
financed programs for dependents. State and local welfare and
Medicaid expenditures would increase both dependency costs,
while expenditures on retirement benefits for nonfederal public
employees would add significantly to the total cost of supporting
the elderly. We are currently in the process of incorporating
these costs in our estimates of the dependency burden. In addition, future research should include private intrafamily and inter-
family expenditures on young and old dependents.

The governmental financing data presented above refer to
programs benefiting the elderly and children, not all of whom fall
into the normal age categories of 65 and over and 18 and
younger. For example, many of the annuitants of federal pensions are below the normal retirement age of 65. At the same
time, children over 18 may, under certain restrictions, continue
to qualify for Social Security and AFDC payments. For analysis
in this paper, the aged dependent population is defined as individuals 65 years and older, while young dependents are represented by the population 18 years of age and less. These age
groupings are frequently used in the literature and for public
policy as the age limits for the dependent population. The average cost of supporting aged dependents in each fiscal year under
the programs previously described is calculated by dividing the
total estimated cost of supporting aged dependents by the number of people 65 and older, while the per-youth expenditure is
attained by dividing the annual cost data by the number of 0–17-
year-olds.

Public expenditures in elementary and secondary schools
amounted to $57 billion in 1973–1974. This represented a per-
student cost of $1,127, which is equal to 24.3 percent of the per
capita DPI. Cost per college student was $2,007, or 43.2 percent
of the per capita DPI. All other direct government expenditures

for youths totaled $13.1 billion, which represented $184 per child under age 18. This cost was equivalent to 3.9 percent of personal per capita disposable income. Thus the estimated dependency cost of supporting youths was $72.9 billion or 7.41 percent of DPI in 1974.

Not every young dependent benefits from these programs; therefore the $184 expenditure per child may be misleading. A more desirable measure might be the compensation per child who is receiving benefits. Such a distinction is important for projections of future dependency costs. For example, the assumption used below that public expenditures for income maintenance and health care benefiting children remain a constant percentage of per capita DPI for each child implies that the proportion of youths receiving such benefits remains constant in the future. If families of various incomes are affected differentially by the trend toward low fertility, the percentage of youths eligible for benefits would change and thereby influence the required level of funding for these programs.

Government programs in support of aged dependents are estimated at $67 billion or $3,071 per individual 65 and older. This level of funding resulted in a public cost of maintaining an elderly dependent amounting to 66.1 percent of per capita DPI. These elderly dependency costs were equal to 6.8 percent of DPI. Therefore in 1974 the public cost of supporting dependents required 14.2 percent of DPI.

To estimate future support patterns, educational enrollment rates are assumed to be constant, while educational expenditure per student and expenditure per dependent for programs other than education are assumed to remain constant percentages of per capita disposable income. In addition, real per capita income is allowed to grow at a constant rate of two percent per year. Population age structures are calculated by using the previously described Bureau of Census (1975) projection of the population Series II. These assumptions also provide for a constant replacement ratio of government benefits to per capita DPI for the elderly, and at the same time entail a constant relative cost of public support for each young dependent enrolled in school.

Within the framework of the above assumptions, the required support patterns until 2050 were calculated. This analysis will ignore any interaction between income and the levels of expenditures on dependents, the composition of dependency costs, and the effect of low fertility rates on the time allocation of individuals. Table 2.7 shows that the percentage of disposable income needed to support publicly financed programs for the aged in the presence of future low fertility rates will rise from 6.8 percent in 1974 to 10.6 percent in 2050. This indicates a rise of over 56 percent in the relative burden on workers to support the elderly. However this increasing burden is offset by a reduction in the proportion of disposable income that is needed to finance the benefits accruing to children. Therefore total dependency cost as a proportion of DPI will rise only two percentage points by 2050. This increase is neither steady nor continuous. In fact, dependency costs will actually decline slightly until the year 2000, because the impact of fewer births will be felt immediately, whereas a significant increase in the proportion of the population over age 65 will occur only after the beginning of the next century. Hogan (1974) has estimated that the total dependency burden will require approximately the same proportion of national income in 2050 that was spent in 1972. The difference between his and our estimates results from Hogan's omission of several of the major support programs for both young and old dependents.

The concluding sections of this paper will focus on (1) the difference in the nature of support payments to the elderly and expenditures used to finance the educational development of children; (2) the possibility that parents are reducing the quantity of children in order to increase their quality, and (3) the potential gain in income with increased female labor force participation as birth rates decline.

Income Effects of Investment in Children vs. Support for the Aged. Most of the expenditures on the elderly could be classified as maintenance costs to society. By this we mean that through its social programs the government is attempting to help the elderly maintain their previous consumption levels and standard of living. Inasmuch as these programs include no investment or capital replacement component, they should have little influence on the future income of the economy. In short, expenditures on the aged represent current consumption and do not increase the productive potential of the economy.

These remarks are not intended to imply that expenditures on the elderly are less desireable than expenditures on children. As previously mentioned, the federal government currently allocates approximately $67 billion to the support of the elderly. Society has chosen to finance these benefits to maximize the aggregate well-being of the population. To the individual elderly dependent, these public funds may represent an investment in his future well-being because they enable the individual to receive proper nourishment and health care, and thus to better enjoy his remaining years. Moreover, part of the expenditure for the elderly represents repayment of monies paid as Social Security taxes while those elderly were themselves working, whereas children have not paid any such taxes.

Society's utility function includes the current and future consumption of all groups. Therefore increasing the level of current consumption by the elderly or any group increases the collective well-being of the nation. In this section, we explain that expenditures on the elderly increase their current consumption and thus increase social utility during this period. In contrast, expenditures on children raise current consumption and through an investment component will increase future consumption. However we do not know the utility that society derives from either expenditure. If the allocation of our resources is currently in equilibrium, then the last dollar spent on the elderly is valued as highly as the last dollar spent on young dependents; with no change in society's preferences or tastes, we would expect a similar allocation of resources in the future.

Much of the expenditures on children directly influence the income-generating capacity of the economy by increasing the stock of human capital. This is clearly the case with educational expenditures, which comprise 84 percent of the total government support for youths. Such spending provides children with the training and skills that enable them to be more productive

Table 2.7 Future Dependency Costs (Billions of Dollars), 1974–2050

Item	1974	1990	2000	2025	2050
Disposable personal income	983.6	1561.6	2,039.1	3,820.0	6,657.7
Expenditures on youths	72.9	95.6	127.1	216.7	373.3
Percent DPI used to finance benefits to children	7.4%	6.1%	6.2%	5.7%	5.6%
Expenditures on elderly	67.0	121.9	157.1	405.2	708.3

Percent DPI used to finance benefits to elderly	6.8%	7.8%	7.7%	10.6%	10.6%
Total dependency costs as percent of DPI	14.2%	13.9%	13.9%	16.3%	16.2%

77

during their work lives and presumably more productive than their parents were. In addition, expenditures on the health and well-being of young individuals in their formative years may also augment their potential contribution to society. Therefore shifts in dependency costs from investment in children to maintenance of the elderly are not without influence upon economic growth. As a result, our assumption that there will be a constant rate of growth in disposable income may be too optimistic.

The relationship between individual educational attainment and earnings is well known. In the aggregate, it implies that increased education and training of members of the labor force increases the rate of growth in income, (Denison, 1968; Jorgenson and Griliches, 1967), that is, investment in youths during this period produces higher income in the post-youth period. Selowsky (1969) shows that growth in income is a function of physical capital accumulation and changes in its productivity, of increases in per capita human capital (greater educational attainment per person), and of changes in the aggregate stock of human capital due to population changes. He found that improvements in the average level of educational attainment in the United States accounted for 0.52 of a percentage point of the annual rate of growth between 1940–1965. Maintaining the same per capita educational levels in the presence of a growing population contributed 0.33 of a percentage point to the growth rate.

We have assumed that the investment rate (as a percentage of per capita DPI) in children remains constant. Thus expenditure per child will rise with increases in income. With low fertility rates, this per capita investment is spread over fewer children and the contribution of maintaining educational standards to the growth in the aggregate stock of human capital and ultimately to the growth in aggregate income will decline. Therefore, if funds that would have been allocated to investment in children in a growing population are used instead to support the aged, future income will decline. Relative support levels of income and benefits will be less because of the change in the composition of dependency costs.

Effects of Demand for Increase in Public Expenditure per Child. Over the past two decades, economists such as Becker (1960) and Schultz (1973) have begun to analyze fertility and expenditures on children within the traditional framework of utility maximization. One of the important findings from this work is the explicit recognition of the substitutability between child quality as represented by expenditure per child and the number of children within a family. In determining their optimum family size, couples must weigh the satisfaction they might derive from children against that received from all other sources and, in addition, they must decide whether having another child would increase their satisfaction more than would increasing the quality of a given number of children.

Becker and Lewis (1973, p. S281) conjecture "that it is plausible to assume that the true income elasticity with respect to quality is substantially larger than that with respect to quantity." The implication of this conjecture is that as incomes rise, parents desire to purchase relatively more quality in their children instead of adding to their family. The relative price of additional children may have been increasing over time, just as the cost of maintaining the same quality of children has been increasing (Heer, 1975). Thus the current low fertility rates may result, in part, from parents choosing to have fewer children of higher quality than in the past.

In our model, a higher quality of children could be attained by raising the expenditures per child or by increasing the enrollment rates. Earlier we assumed that government educational expenditures per child would remain a fixed proportion of per capita DPI. If this level of spending is raised in response to voter pressure, the dependency costs of providing education to youths would, of course, be higher than the estimates in Table 2.7. Similarly, higher enrollment would mean that a higher percentage of the DPI would be needed to finance the educational system.

Kreps and Clark (1975) have shown that, while the enrollment rates of individuals over 18 have declined somewhat since the late 1960s, the proportion of youths under 18 who are still in school has continued to increase. Enrollment rates for children 6–15 have remained relatively constant near 98 percent, and the rates for youths 16–17 have been relatively stable since the mid-60s, in the neighborhood of 88 percent. The rapid expansion of public and private kindergartens and preschools has produced significant increases in the enrollment rates for children three to five years old. The proportion of three- and four-year-olds attending schools rose from 9.5 percent in 1964 to 28.8 percent in 1974, while the rates for five-year-olds increased from 68.5 percent in 1964 to 84.1 percent in 1973 (School enrollment, 1975; National Center for Education Statistics, 1975). Levitan and Alderman (1975) estimated that approximately $3.5 billion was spent by governmental units to finance child care and educational expenditures for preschool-age children.

As a result of the increases in the enrollment rates and higher expenditures per student, governmental expenditures on elementary and secondary schools rose as a percentage of disposable personal income from 6.09 percent in 1967 to 6.24 percent in 1974, despite a reduction in the percentage of the population that was less than 18 years old. One set of projections forecasts that the enrollment rates of preschool-age children will continue to rise. Froomkin, Endriss & Stump (1971) estimated that by the end of the 1970s, 55 percent of all three-year-olds, 77 percent of four-year-olds, and virtually all the five-year-olds will be attending school. As these enrollment rates continue to increase, our estimates of the percentage of DPI needed to finance programs for young dependents will understate the future costs. Therefore future demand for public expenditures to produce children of higher quality will reduce any potential trade-off in dependency costs associated with low fertility rates.

Effects of Demand for Improvements in Programs Serving the Elderly. A similar demand by the aged may be in the offing as they attempt to improve the relative quality of life in retirement. The replacement ratio for the average beneficiary under Social Security has remained relatively stable over the past 25 years. Increases in the proportion of national income required to finance this program have resulted primarily from the expanded coverage (beneficiaries as a percentage of the aged) of the system. Since the system is now almost universal, future increases of this type will not occur. However pressure may grow to raise the replacement ratio. Such increases would have a significant impact on the level of support required to finance this program (Clark, 1975). In addition, there has been a rapid expansion in recent years of Medicare, Medicaid, food stamps, and the other income security programs. Continued improvements in these programs would raise the percentage of DPI necessary to finance them. Thus future improvements in the relative position of the aged will require a greater proportion of the nation's output than we estimate in Table 2.7.

Effects of Changes in the Labor Force Participation Rate of Women. A common argument is that lower fertility will permit greater female participation in market activity and thus increase the number of workers and mitigate each worker's burden. Since child care is a major home-produced service which historically has required a relatively large input of the mother's time, the presence of small children lowers the labor force participation rates and hours of work of mothers. In 1974 the market activity rate of married women with children under six was 34.4 percent, while that of wives with no children under age 18 was 43 percent. The most significant difference, however, was between women with children under age three, who had a labor force participation rate of 31 percent, and those with children aged six to 17, whose participation rate was 51.2 percent (Hayghe, 1975; U.S. Department of Labor, 1973).

An implication of the above data is that children may have a two-stage impact on the labor market activity of their mothers. While children are less than three years old, there is a significant reduction in labor force participation by mothers, because the family's burden of child supervision is borne primarily by the wife. But once children reach age six, the school system provides virtually free child care while income demands on the family may be increasing. Within this context, women with children 6–17 have a higher propensity to be in the market than any other group of married women. Thus the total influence of children on the working life of married women is not as unambiguous as the effect of young children.

Over the past decade and a half, labor force participation by women with children of all ages has increased significantly. Since 1960, the participation rate of mothers with children under three has more than doubled, and by 1974 there was little difference between the market activity of women with children three to five years of age and those with no children under age 18 (Hayghe, 1974; U.S. Department of Labor, 1973). Continuation of these trends could soon make the work patterns for women with small children similar to those of all married women. For example, in 1960 the labor force participation rate of women with children under the age of three was 44 percent of the rate of married women with no children under the age of 18. By 1974, however, the market activity rate of women with such children was 72 percent of that of the group with no children under the age of 18. Therefore the future gain in labor force participation due to low fertility rates (which imply fewer women with young children) may be insignificant in magnitude and considerably less important than the predicted increase due to the continued upward movement of labor force participation rates among women of all groups.

In addition, one must not equate the gain in income due to the increased market activity of women with increases in aggregate utility or well-being. These new entrants into the labor force were previously allocating their time to other pursuits. Women not in the labor force contribute to their family's welfare by performing many household tasks. The lack of reliable data on the value of household production often means that this source of wealth to the family is overlooked.

One study of the value of nonmarket activity (Sirageldin, 1969, p. 53) stated that "in 1964 the average value of unpaid output for the American family is estimated at $3,929 or about 50 percent of its disposable income." Therefore the true gain to increased female labor force participation would be the rise in measured income less any loss in nonmarket production that occurs when the woman has fewer hours of home time. An additional caveat is that much of the time of women outside the labor market is spent in child rearing, i.e., a form of investment in the child (Dugan, 1969). Thus any reallocation of this time may imply a reduction in the society's investment in human capital. Many services which support the aged are also provided by women in their nonmarket time. As a result, the movement of women into the labor force may lower the well-being of the elderly.

Composition of Labor Force and Factors Affecting the Income and Participation of Older Workers. To show the future course of the proportion of the population expected to be in the labor force, Table 8 shows the Department of Labor projections of labor force participation to 1990. According to these projections, overall labor force participation on the part of those 16 and over will rise from 60.3 percent in 1970 to 61.5 percent by 1990. Although a slight decline is expected in male labor force participation, an appreciable increase is predicted in female labor force participation (Johnston, 1973). Significant decreases are expected, however, in the market activity rates of the male population aged 55–64 and over 64. Given labor force participation at the rates projected in Table 2.8, increases in the burden on the working population in supporting dependents will not be caused by shifts or declines in the proportion of the population that is in the labor force.

Labor force projections are subject to increasing uncertainty because of possible changes both in the value attached by potential workers to work and in the income and work conditions to which potential workers must respond. Increases in retirement income, together with reduction in the age at which such income may begin, tend to discourage work, whereas inflation, by eroding the purchasing power of prospective retirement income, encourages labor force participation because continuation of earnings provides the primary assurance against pronounced shrinkage in real income. With over half the nation's voting power in the hands of persons under 45, there is a political limit to the degree of increase in Social Security taxation that will be tolerated. There are also corresponding limits to the degree to which contractual money incomes subject to erosion by inflation

Table 2.8 Labor Force Participation Rates, 1970, 1980, 1990 (in Percentage of Age Category Population)

Age	Male			Female		
	1970	1980	1990	1970	1980	1990
16 and over	79.2	78.0	78.4	42.8	45.0	45.9
16–19	57.5	56.0	55.4	43.7	45.5	47.0
20–24	85.1	83.0	82.1	57.5	63.4	66.2
25–34	95.0	94.6	94.4	44.8	50.2	51.5
35–44	95.7	95.1	94.7	50.9	53.2	55.2
45–54	92.9	91.9	91.5	54.0	56.2	58.0
55–59	88.0	86.6	85.9	48.4	51.2	52.9
60–64	73.6	70.3	68.9	35.6	37.5	38.8
65–69	40.7	35.5	33.6	16.4	16.5	16.4
70+	16.9	12.7	11.0	5.0	4.9	4.6

Source: U.S. Department of Labor (1975, p. 309).

can be augmented. Even in the absence of inflation, retired persons may experience what amounts to erosion of their relative income positions if the average worker income should rise, say, two percent annually, because retirees are unlikely to share equally in this increase.

When the demand for labor is not very elastic and when new entrants into the labor force are more skilled or lower priced than those already in the labor force, some members of the labor force are likely to be displaced. This appears to have happened in the past to older male workers upon the entry of better educated younger workers. Microeconomic barriers to increases in employment may also limit the fraction of those in the latter stages of work life who can find and maintain employment, thereby strengthening incentives to withdraw from the labor force. Among these barriers are uniform wage rates imposed by governments and trade unions, together with other expensive conditions attached to employing potential workers. Given these conditions, it may be profitable for management to economize in the use of labor and to avoid risks associated with hiring older workers.

Two factors relating to future dependency costs have been purposely omitted from our discussion. First, we have considered only governmental expenditures. Any family with children necessarily reallocates its purchase of goods and services. Cain (1971) estimated the cost of a child to a four-person family earning $9,000 annually. The present value of the "total costs to the parents of a child, including the dominant component of time foregone, is around $31,000" (p. 412). As we all know, the family bears these costs by adjusting its other purchases and allocation of time. In the future, will this money be available to support the aged? To the extent that the government can increase the tax burden, some of these funds will be available. However this does not imply that any family would be as satisfied with spending money on its own child as with having the same amount transferred by the government to the elderly. Secondly, we have set the maximum age of young dependents at 18 years. Because of this age limitation, most of the cost of financing higher education is omitted from our dependency costs. The inclusion of expenditures on colleges and universities would raise measured support costs and might also influence the trend of these costs.

SUMMARY

The initial section of this paper reviewed the anticipated changes in the composition of the dependency ratio implied by the continuation of low rates of fertility. These projections show that, under replacement level fertility, the proportion of population 65 and over rises from 10 percent in 1975 to 16 percent in 2050, while the percentage aged 0–17 falls from 31 to 25 percent. Thus, in the future the working population will be called upon to support more older dependents but fewer young dependents.

Since the total dependency ratio is not expected to change significantly under these conditions, the future of the dependency burden on the working population depends on the relative costs of supporting young versus old dependents. At current levels of financing, governmental expenditures per elderly dependent are considerably greater than similar expenditures per young dependent. Therefore the shift from young dependents to elderly dependents will necessitate an increase in the dependency burden. Within the framework of the model described in this chapter, the required level of governmental supports increases from 14.2 percent of disposable personal income in 1974 to 16.2 percent in 2050.

In addition to the greater dependency burden, the future allocation of support costs will have an impact on the level of income and the rate of economic growth. The reason for this interaction between changing dependency costs and growth is that expenditures on youths represent, to a large degree, investment in human capital, and therefore they influence society's future earnings. Expenditures on the aged are, however, primarily maintenance costs and do not influence the productive potential of the economy. Thus the reallocation of funds from programs for young dependents to programs for the elderly may lower future income.

Low fertility may influence more women to enter the labor market and thereby augment national income. Recent projections, however, indicate that the total increase in female labor force participation by 1990 will only slightly outweigh the expected decline in the market activity of males. We also point out that the gap between labor force involvement of women with children and those without has been narrowing over the past decade. One must also remember that the gain in income due to women moving into the labor force does not represent an equivalent gain in welfare, because a drop in home-produced services would be expected. There is a clear trade-off of support costs as society is required to support fewer young dependents and more aged ones. However an elderly dependent costs the government more to maintain than does a young dependent. Therefore the trade-off is not dollar for dollar as the composition of the dependency ratio changes. The primary conclusion of this paper must be that the continuation of low fertility rates will probably require an increase in the publicly financed dependency burden on the working population.

REFERENCES

Becker, G. An economic analysis of fertility. In *Demographic and economic change in developed countries.* Princeton: Princeton University Press, 1960.

Becker, G., & Lewis, G. On the interaction between quantity and quality of children. *Journal of Political Economy,* 1973, *81*(2, Part II), S279–299.

Cain, G. Issues in the economics of a population policy for the United States. *American Economic Review,* 1971, *61*(2), 408–417.

Clark, R. Age structure changes and intergenerational transfers of income. Unpublished monograph. Duke University, 1975.

Coale, A. J. Alternative paths to a stationary population. In *Demographic and social aspects of population growth, I.* C. F. Westoff & R. Parke, Jr. (Eds.), Washington, D.C.: U.S. Commission on Population Growth, 1972.

Coale, A. J., & Demeny, P. *Regional model life tables and stable populations.* Princeton: Princeton University Press, 1966.

Council of Economic Advisers. *Economic Report of the President: 1976.* Washington, D.C.: U.S. Government Printing Office, 1976.

Denison, E. *Why growth rates differ.* Washington, D.C.: The Brookings Institution, 1968.

Dugan, D. The impact of parental and educational investments upon student achievement. *Proceedings of the American Statistical Association, Social Statistics Section,* 1969, pp. 138–148.

Fogel, W. A. Immigrant Mexicans and the U.S. labor force. *Monthly Labor Review,* 1975, *98*(5), 44–46.

Froomkin, J., Endriss, J. R., & Stump, R. *Population, enrollment, and costs of public elementary and secondary education 1975–1976 and 1980–1981: A report to the President's commission of school finance.* Washington, D.C.: The President's Commission on School Finance, 1971.

Hayghe, H. Marital and family characteristics of the labor force in March 1973. *Monthly Labor Review,* 1974, *97*(4), 21–27.

Hayghe, H. Marital and family characteristics of workers. *Monthly Labor Review,* 1975, *98*(1), 60–64.

Heer, D. *Society and population* (2nd ed.). Englewood Cliffs, N.J.: Prentice-Hall, 1975.

Hogan, T. D. Implications of Population Stationarity for the Social Security System. *Social Science Quarterly,* 1974, June, 151–158.

Johnston, D. F. Labor force projections to 1990. *Monthly Labor Review,* 1973, *96*(7), 3–13.

Jorgenson, D., & Griliches, Z. The explanation of productivity change. *Review of Economics Studies,* 1967, *34*(99), 249–283.

Kreps, J., & Clark, R. *Sex, age and work.* Baltimore: Johns Hopkins University Press, 1975.

Levitan, S., & Alderman, K. *Child care and ABC's too.* Baltimore: Johns Hopkins University Press, 1975.

Metropolitan Life Insurance Company. Potential gains in longevity after midlife. *Statistical Bulletin,* 1975, *56*(9).

National Center for Education Statistics. *Digest of Educational Statistics* (1974 ed.). U.S. Department of Health, Education and Welfare. Washington, D.C.: U.S. Government Printing Office, 1975.

Office of Management and Budget. *Special Analysis: Budget of the United States Government, Fiscal Year 1976.* Washington, D.C.: U.S. Government Printing Office, 1975.

Piore, M. J. Impact of immigration on the labor force. *Monthly Labor Review,* 1975, *98*(5), 41–43.

School enrollment—Social and economic characteristics of students: October 1974. *Current Population Reports* (Series P-20, No. 286). Washington, D.C.: U.S. Government Printing Office, 1975.

Schultz, T. W. *Economics of the family: Marriage, children and human capital.* Chicago: University of Chicago Press, 1973.

Selowsky, M. On the measurement of education's contribution to growth. *Quarterly Journal of Economics,* 1969, *83*(3), 449–463.

Sirageldin, I. A. *Non-market components of national income.* Ann Arbor, Michigan: Institute for Social Research, 1969.

United Nations. The aging of populations and its economic and social implications. *Population Studies,* 1956, *26,* 27–29.

U.S. Department of Commerce, Bureau of the Census. Projections of the population of the United States: 1975–2050. *Current Population Reports* (Series P-25, No. 601). Washington, D.C.: U.S. Government Printing Office, 1975.

U.S. Department of Labor. *Dual Careers 2.* Manpower Research Monograph No. 21. Washington, D.C.: U.S. Government Printing Office, 1973.

U.S. Department of Labor. *Manpower Report of the President.* Washington, D.C.: U.S. Government Printing Office, 1975.

U.S. News & World Report, January 26, 1976, pp. 84–85.

-Part II-

WORK:
ITS POTENTIAL ROLE

The desirability and practicality of more freedom of choice in allocating time for work, education, and leisure is the theme of the next two chapters. In them, economist Malcolm Morrison and training specialist R. Meredith Belbin examine ways in which alternatives could be offered, suggesting the value of increased flexibility not only for the individual, but for the population at large, who will be asked to support an increasing number of future retirees.

Morrison's chapter discusses the various economic forces which are inducing workers to opt for early retirement, and which have prevented the emergence of policies allowing more freedom of choice for older workers. Creating real choice, he believes, involves more than just devising special programs for the older population group; effective programs should encompass all workers. He cites many examples, including two far-reaching proposals by Gosta Rehn and Jule Sugarman. Rehn's proposal calls for creating an integrated insurance system for transferring income between different periods of life. Each person would have the right to draw on his or her account for various purposes, including periods of leisure and education. Under Sugarman's decennial sabbatical plan, a portion of each person's earnings would be set aside for each of nine consecutive years, and in every tenth year the accumulated sum would finance a year of income without employment, thus providing opportunities for education or leisure and at the same time reducing overall unemployment through sharing of work.

In Chapter 4, Meredith Belbin notes the wide variation in retirement age among European countries—a variation not tied to the wealth of the countries—as well as the strong trend toward decreased work activity by older men. He points out the interest shown by many Europeans in improving retirement policies, and is reasonably optimistic that efforts by individual European countries will produce models which may be adapted elsewhere. In France, for example, employers are now required to contribute a set percentage of their wage bill for a nationwide system of lifelong education. Workers of any age have a right to take paid leave for further education and training. Other European countries are focusing on ways to foster gradual retirement. A proposal currently attracting much attention in England calls for providing social security and occupational pensions at half-rates until age 70 (except for those who are disabled), thus stimulating older people to continue to work on a part-time basis. Private industry's reluctance to employ part-time workers might be overcome through tax incentives—including the waiver of social security payments for older employees—reinforced by a tough age-discrimination law. The scene might then be set, Belbin suggests, for managers to work out the most effective way of utilizing older workers' skills.

Morrison and Belbin suggest a number of innovative ideas, but neither spell out in specific detail how the ideas they describe might be meshed into the present U.S. pension and educational arrangements. We stand in need of more information on how European experiments are working, as well as specific and detailed proposals for how the U.S. system might be modified to provide a greater choice in allocation of time between work, leisure, and education.

-3-

Flexible Distribution of Work, Leisure, and Education: Potentials for the Aging

Malcolm H. Morrison

Work which is indispensable for man's survival, no longer takes up his entire life as was once the case. It is precisely a balance between working time and non-working time which is one of the major problems today since as Pierre Naville said it is "the free use of his time . . . which gives a real price to man's existence." (Maric, 1973, p. 17)

Only a short time ago, the possibility of significant individual variations in the use of time throughout life seemed an impossible dream. However, improving economic conditions now make possible the serious consideration of practical proposals for greater flexibility in the use of time throughout life. Because of the changing economic environment

social policies which encourage the adoption of new ways of making use of time should be examined in greater depth so that the advantages and disadvantages of various experiments can be compared, e.g. variable timetable or shift work, four or five-day week, holidays divided over different times of the year or a single long holiday, early or postponed retirement (in whole or in part) prolonged studies and training for the young or continuing training at recurrent periods throughout life. (de Chalendar, 1973, p. 5)

This chapter urges the consideration of approaches which would increase opportunities for individuals to choose between greater income through employment and/or more time off from regular work at older ages. Such approaches should be designed to encourage greater freedom of choice in the distribution of leisure time, and thus to bring more flexibility to working life.

In creating opportunities for greater choice for older workers, the constraints of existing public and private retirement pension arrangements must be recognized. However the formulation of new alternatives must not be limited by such constraints, because with the development of new conceptualizations of the work life, such constraints may not prove to be significant barriers to innovation.

New and flexible approaches for the allocation of time for work, leisure, and education throughout life are now being developed in many countries, and specific reforms have been adopted in some instances. Recent concern with increasing the flexible distribution of work, education, and leisure results from numerous social and economic developments in industrialized nations. These include shorter annual working hours, longer periods of education, improved retirement conditions, increasing employment of women who need to combine income producing and home work, problems of industrial relations fostered by rigid working conditions, problems of employment of older workers and their transition to retirement, and development of programs of further training and education during the working years.

Most countries retain the economic objective of full utilization of the labor force and the social objective of providing the worker with as much choice as possible in allocating both working and nonworking time. Economic and social systems are continually being modified to attain these objectives. Recent changes in economic conditions (including higher levels of unemployment and concurrent inflation/recession), and in social preferences (including worker demands for increasing amounts of nonwork time) have stimulated discussion of new variations in working and leisure time patterns. Further exploration of new approaches to the organization and distribution of time throughout life is long overdue in the United States.

As part of these economic and social changes, the development of new patterns of distribution of work, leisure, and education in the life cycle is anticipated. Some early changes are already occurring; much more will change in the future. We have the opportunity to shape these changes in directions that conform to our economic and social objectives. Whether we do so will depend upon a convergence of economic and social thought and a willingness to experiment with new approaches to the utilization and organization of time.

If we assume that economic growth will continue, the most fundamental question for the future is: *To what extent will people prefer more leisure time to more real income* (which involves more work)? Undoubtedly preferences will vary between countries and will depend in part upon standard of living, economic development, availability of employment, options for use of leisure time, national institutionalized practices, and cultural traditions.

Numerous factors influence the amount of time spent working during the life span. Among the more important are (1) time used for training and education prior to regular employment; (2) time used for education and training during the years of regular employment; (3) length of time spent at work (working day, week, and year); (4) duration of holidays; (5) periods spent away from work during the worklife; and (6) the time of retirement from regular work.

In approaching the specific problems of workers as they age, two major goals have emerged: adequate financial benefits for the support of persons who have retired from regular employment, and greater flexibility in the aging worker's choice of when to retire, partially or fully, from regular employment. These two objectives are not in conflict. It certainly appears that as the levels of retirement income benefits increase, the proportion of older workers who choose to retire also gradually increases, but a certain number of persons remain motivated to continue regular employment. This occurs if the opportunity to continue working is an important social and economic objective. Increasing the financial benefits for persons who choose or are forced to retire is also an important objective. These two objectives can and should be pursued simultaneously.

When considering new patterns for the use of time it is important to approach the problem broadly. The *quantity* of time spent at work or at leisure is not the most important measure of flexibility. The value attached to time depends largely on the *quality* of work and the quality of leisure. Social policy should be concerned with improving the quality of these experiences and with increasing the available freedom of choice regarding the amounts of time spent in these pursuits. The fundamental problem of new patterns in work time should not be treated as an isolated issue. It is directly involved with such areas as (1) economic growth, (2) choices between greater income or greater leisure for the individual, (3) the type of growth preferred by the social system, (4) employment and working conditions, and (5) education and training.

Creating more freedom of choice for older workers involves more than devising special programs for this population group. Prevalent economic and social trends in each country must be taken into account. Proposals for change must not be restricted to the aged alone, but rather must include all segments of the population. Given the trend of early retirement, it may be essential to develop a new view of the worklife which incorporates the flexible distribution of employment, leisure, and education, if actual freedom of choice is ever to be available to most aging workers.

Since 1900 the number and proportion of older persons in the U.S. population has been growing at an increasing rate. Projections indicate that increases will continue and will be of major significance in the early and middle years of the 21st century. These projections and resultant dependency ratios are discussed in chapters by Havighurst, Clark and Spengler, and Munnell, and will not be restated here. However it is important to point out that the substantial increase in the number and proportion of older persons will necessitate changes in the methods of providing economic support to the retired and in the options provided to those who wish to continue some form of regular employment. In short, demographic change implies both problems and possibilities for the future. Although we can anticipate a continuation of the current early retirement trend at least in the near future, older persons in the first part of the next century may want more freedom of choice as to their patterns of work, leisure, and education. Certainly their numbers will be sufficient to influence social change toward such an objective.

THE U.S. ECONOMY: 1970–1990

An examination of trends in economic development and their effects on employment and working time provides information useful in assessing potentials for change in the distribution of time through the life cycle.

Since the end of World War II, the overall performance of the United States economy has been excellent in comparison to earlier historical periods. Since 1950 the gross national product has risen dramatically, as have personal consumption expenditures, gross domestic private investment, and government expenditures. During this same period civilian employment also has grown significantly, and through 1974 unemployment had not remained high (above 6 percent) for any lengthy period of time.

Despite this economic growth, several serious problems have continued to elude solution. Among these are continuing inflation and the achievement of the goals of full employment and price stability. To better understand the prospects of these areas we should review economic performance since 1969, because some developments since that time have led to certain unique economic problems which affect today's elderly (Pechman, 1976).

Shortly after taking office in 1969, President Nixon and his economic advisors concluded that the most serious problem then facing the economy was inflation and that the way to control it was by reducing the rate of growth in demand through fiscal and monetary policies. The administration responded to the problem by first tightening the money supply and restricting available credit. Later, the money supply was increased and wage and price controls were implemented. In early 1973 price controls were eased, and by mid-1974 they were eliminated completely. Presumably the change in policy was an attempt to allow market forces to operate freely, on the assumption that the overall expansion would continue as would the trends of lower unemployment and inflation rates.

Unfortunately these results did not occur. In 1974 wholesale and consumer prices rose more than 10 percent for the year, and wages increased rapidly in 1974–1975 in an effort to keep up with prices. Unemployment reached very high levels in 1974, 1975, and 1976. Thus, since 1969 inflation has continued to be a serious problem and has not abated even with increased unemployment. It now seems that inflation results in subsequent wage increases irrespective of unemployment. Moreover, even if the Federal Reserve does not loosen the supply of money in response to higher prices, the effect seems to be not reduced inflation, but increased unemployment.

Recently there has been some evidence of an upturn in the economy with increased consumer demand and increased business investment and production. Unemployment has shown signs of abating during recent months. However the wage-price cycle is continuing and inflation is proceeding at about a six percent annual rate. These facts mean that the underlying problems identified in 1969 are continuing and that neither fiscal nor monetary policies have thus far been able to effectively combat the problem. Thus we are faced with the prospect of continuing high unemployment and inflation as we approach the 1980s.

Effects of Unemployment on Options for Distribution of Work, Leisure, and Education. While periods of strong demand may reduce unemployment, the wage-price cycle may fuel inflation and result in continued attempts by the government to cool the economy, which could increase unemployment again. Unless the government moves in the direction of wage and price guidelines or controls, the economic environment will continue to be characterized by forced leisure because of unemployment and the restrictive monetary policies used in attempts to control inflation. Neither of these conditions is particularly conducive to the development of a more flexible distribution of work, leisure, and education. In fact, workers may be forced to choose higher income rather than decreased working time in order to keep up with conditions of inflation. Firms may be reluctant to experiment with alternative choices for the distribution of time because of monetary constraints and the desire to limit the work force. And continuing high rates of unemployment may result in earlier retirement for older workers with few real options for gradual or later retirement.

In the United States, where both gains in productivity and increases in the labor force are likely, particularly strong efforts to achieve a high growth rate are essential if relatively full employment is to be maintained. Gains in productivity not accompanied by higher growth would result in levels of unemployment which would be an ever increasing burden on those remaining employed. Therefore a simple reduction in the number of persons employed is not really a feasible approach to reallocating time, because those not working would have to be supported by those working (with significant effects on income). Moreover, such support would be at economic levels too low to allow for active leisure pursuits, which often involve relatively high expense. New approaches to the allocation of time for work, leisure, and education should be implemented without resorting to the creation of "forced leisure" because of high rates of unemployment.

Alternatives for reallocating time would be best developed in environments where economic growth is sufficient to generate employment for most of the working-age population. In such settings meaningful reforms for reallocation of time—which would not involve artificial leisure due to unemployment and its concomitant income support problems—could be achieved more easily.

It is important to recognize that economic conditions are not immutable and that they are not the only determinants of whether new approaches are developed and implemented. Rather, they constitute a fundamental part of the environment in which innovations must be launched. Therefore recognition of economic conditions can be helpful in assessing the probable acceptance of and support for various proposals for change.

WORKING TIME AND PREFERENCES
FOR LEISURE VS. INCOME

For about the last 10 years the actual length of time worked by wage earners has been falling in most European countries and in the United States. The average work week in the U.S. was 38.6 hours in 1960 and 37.4 hours in 1970 (Table 3.1). While the number of hours spent working has been decreasing in many countries, other factors have also acted to shorten the overall length of working life. Two of the most important factors are longer school attendance and/or longer periods of initial vocational training and earlier retirement encouraged by certain "flexible" retirement provisions of public and private pension systems. As the length of working time has decreased, various patterns of preference for the distribution of time have emerged in different countries. Some of these recent patterns have been reported by the Organization for Economic Cooperation and Development (de Chalendar, 1973):

- *United States, Australia*—preference for shorter working day or week rather than for longer vacation or lower retirement age
- *Canada*—preference for longer annual vacation and same working week
- *France*—preference for additional training during working life and lower retirement age
- *Netherlands*—preference for longer period of initial training and lower retirement age
- *Germany*—preference for lowering retirement age, shortening work week, and lengthening annual vacation
- *Sweden*—preference for lengthening vacation and shortening work week rather than lowering retirement age

The trend is clearly in the direction of a shorter working life during the next two decades. It is striking, however, that only a small portion of the significant productivity gains in the past 25 years have reduced working time. In the United States, for example, the need for increased income has been so great that the

Table 3.1 Hours in the Working Week, Nonagricultural Sectors[a]

Country	1960	1969	1970
Federal Republic of Germany [c,d]	45.3	44.0	44.2
Australia [c,e]			
Men	—	43.6	—
Women	—	39.4	—
Spain [b,f,g]	43.6	44.1	44.1
United States [c]	38.6	37.7	37.4
France [b]	46.5	45.9	45.6
Ireland [b,h]	45.5	—	—
Italy [b,h,i]	—	7.82	—
Japan [b,g]	46.8	43.9	44.5
United Kingdom [b,e,j]			
Men	48.0	46.5	—
Women	40.5	38.1	—

[a] Unless otherwise stated in the footnotes, the figures given in this table cover the following branches of economic activity: mining and quarrying; manufacturing industry; building and construction; commerce; transport; warehousing and communications; services.
[b] Hours actually worked.
[c] Hours paid.
[d] Excluding commerce and transport.

[e] Adults only.
[f] Including clerical staff.
[g] Excluding transport. 1960 excludes commerce.
[h] Excluding commerce and transport.
[i] Per day.
[j] Excluding coalmining, commerce and British railways.
Source: Maric (1973).

number of hours worked decreased only slightly during the 1960–1970 decade (Moore & Hedges, 1971). Recent serious inflation certainly has increased the need for more income, and workers' preferences for higher earnings (rather than more leisure) are constantly expressed.

A major question for the future is whether the desire for more income will continue to be so much greater than the desire for leisure or time off from work. As is true with most of the issues concerning flexibility in the allocation of time, there are no firm data that can answer this question. Although some of the reductions in "standard" and "actual" hours of work are being absorbed by increases in "work-related" time (such as travel time and continued training and education), the desire for more leisure time will certainly increase as we approach the year 2000. (Kahn & Wiener, 1967). Surveys conducted in a number of countries show that as income rises, the propensity toward leisure is higher than the preference for increased earnings (Rustant, 1973).

It is important to note, however, that leisure and recreation taking place in the home are usually inexpensive, whereas other forms of leisure such as vacations, travel, sports, and hobbies tend to be relatively costly. The worker who desires the more costly forms of leisure will therefore have to modify his desire to work fewer hours in order to acquire the resources necessary to support such recreational activities.

Preferences for the shortening of work time will continue to differ from country to country. Such preferences are subject to change, however, and current preferences cannot be assumed to represent any long-term trends. We do know that we are moving toward a reduction in working time which will take a variety of forms including shorter work weeks, longer vacations, more holidays, earlier retirement, and longer periods of training. In view of the fact that both a shorter work life and a continually increasing life expectancy are likely prospects, the question can be raised whether the older worker should be encouraged to stop regular work at an earlier age or whether other alternatives such as continued training, retraining, or part-time work for the older employee should be encouraged to avoid a prolonged retirement.

Periods of Life and Options in Old Age. Although any division of life into stages is arbitrary, consideration of new alternatives for flexible distribution of time can only proceed within a framework which emphasizes the most prominent features of various periods of the life span. From this point of view, the major question to be raised is to what extent the distribution of time for study (initial education), for paid employment, household, and family activities (the working years), and for increased leisure (the retirement years), can be improved for each individual.

These divisions are somewhat arbitrary. Young persons often take jobs before completing their initial education; further training and education often occur during the working years; many persons, especially married women, leave paid employment for prolonged periods during the working years; and near the conclusion of working life, the transition to retirement may be gradual with some paid work taking place both before and after retirement. Although there are numerous aspects of flexibility during the formative years, (e.g. compulsory schooling and structure of education systems, vocational training, apprenticeship, and transition to work), and during the working years (e.g. weekly hours of work, scheduling of work, overtime, secondary jobs, distribution of hours of work, shift work, variable work schedules, part-time employment, time off for vacation periods, and for further education and training), the focus of our concern is on the later working years which are commonly called the retirement years.

In recent years the practice of abrupt retirement from regular employment has been subject to increasing criticism. The desirability or necessity of ending work suddenly at a predetermined age, irrespective of individual work capacities, abilities, and desires, is now subject to serious question. *It is our view that mature and older workers should have increased opportunities for choice between leisure and work as they approach retirement. The creation of options for such flexibility reflects an appreciation of changes in working capacity with age and also recognizes that older persons are often reluctant to make sudden drastic changes in their styles of life.*

It has been suggested that there is a general desire for individual flexibility in choosing a retirement age, including both early and later retirement. In addition, suggestions have been made (1) that retirement should occur as a transitional process, with workers being allowed to taper off regular work both before and after the so-called usual retirement age; (2) that the possibility of temporary retirement should be introduced whereby a period of retirement might be followed by a return to work; and (3) that regular full-time work beyond the usual retirement age should be made a real option for older workers (de Chalendar, 1973). What the above recommendations really argue for is the introduction of much greater flexibility into the retirement process. While such an objective is laudable in and of itself, it will be difficult to implement. Any innovations in flexibility must be introduced into an environment heavily influenced by an interrelated set of factors: the provisions of current pension systems; the responses of workers to these provisions; and general economic conditions that affect the availability of employment and the willingness of private and public organizations to allow for various flexible innovations.

Basically, there are four major options available to older workers: early retirement from regular employment; retirement at the "regular" age mandated by various pension systems; transitional retirement (gradual reduction of work, possibly both before and after retirement); and continuation of regular full-time employment beyond the "normal" retirement age.

Older persons cannot exercise a completely free choice of options as they approach retirement. The choices which can be made are shaped by pension system regulations, the individual's own thoughts about the best course of action (based on his income, health, attitude, and personal requirements), the state of the labor market, and employer and trade union policies and practices. There has been interest in the employment of older workers, and various manpower policies and programs have been recommended to encourage such employment. However in many cases these approaches have not been based upon an analysis of (1) the provisions of pension systems (which might provide incentives or disincentives for flexibility); (2) the response of older workers to these provisions; (3) labor market constraints; or (4) business or trade union policy constraints. The development of realistic proposals to encourage greater flexibility requires consideration of the above factors.

The major goal of a constructive manpower policy is providing an opportunity for each individual to choose to utilize his or her ability productively in the national economy. Pension and personnel policies and regulations and rules that *encourage* the removal of individuals from the labor force do not accomplish this goal. If current retirement programs are encouraging the development of idleness among a growing "young-old" population and are resulting in increasing economic hardship for such persons, these programs cannot be viewed as satisfactory. Evidence exists that many older workers have a limited understanding of what their economic situation in retirement will be and often retire without realizing either that they will have insufficient income or that they will be unable to reverse their retirement decision, because finding regular employment after retirement is extremely difficult. Little is being done to remedy this serious problem (Morrison, 1975).

THE IMPACT OF RETIREMENT PLANS ON EMPLOYMENT OF THE AGED

Concern has been growing over the fiscal integrity of both the Social Security system and private pension programs. The future shift in the age composition of the population will result in an increasing burden on the active labor force to support a larger number and proportion of older persons. The financial burden on workers could be significantly reduced through the adoption of policies which would encourage people to remain in the labor force beyond the normally accepted retirement age. If even a reasonable proportion of future older workers continues regular

employment, the long-range potential actuarial deficit in the Social Security program could be virtually eliminated.

> The most significant social trend causing higher than necessary
> social security costs in the next century is this trend toward earlier
> retirement. If we could reverse this trend and have *greater* labor
> force participation among older people in the next century than we
> have today, there could be a significant saving for social security
> over what is currently estimated. There may well be a question
> whether a policy of earlier and earlier retirement makes sense—
> either for the individual or for society—when one considers the
> probability of more older people living somewhat longer and with
> a high proportion of those in the younger part of the aged popula-
> tion being in reasonably good health. One quite possible and highly
> rational response to the change in the age distribution of the popu-
> lation now being predicted would be for society to employ a higher
> proportion of older people (Ball, 1975, p. 16).

This type of policy would tend to reduce the cost of private
pensions as well, because the major determinant of pension costs
is the proportion of the aged group which is retired and thus
drawing pension benefits, rather than that which is employed and
not drawing benefits.

National Social Insurance. The United States has a national
social insurance (Social Security) program—old age, survivors,
disability, and health insurance—which covers nearly all employees and self-employed persons in the country, and a special
system for railroad employees (separate retirement programs
cover federal government employees and some state and local
government employees). The program is financed from contributions payable by employees and employers without any governmental contribution. Old age pensions are normally payable
in full at age 65 but may be optionally claimed at age 62 with a
reduction in benefits. If workers postpone retirement beyond age
65, their benefits are increased 1/12 of one percent for each
month between ages 65 and 72 for which no benefits are received. Retired workers *under age 72* who are entitled to monthly
cash benefits under the program are affected by an *earnings test*
provision in the law if they receive income from employment in
excess of specific monthly and yearly amounts. The earnings test

provision is based upon the principle that social insurance pension benefits should be paid only to those who suffer loss of employment income, but at the same time should not discourage limited supplementation of income for "retired" persons wishing to pursue some work.

In a sense, the government through Social Security has initiated a flexible retirement approach which allows retirement as early as age 62 for both men and women. This option has had significant effects on the size and age composition of the labor force, and in fact, age 62 may be becoming the de facto retirement age in the United States.

Private Pensions. In the United States there exists a wide variety of private pension plans. In most cases private pensions constitute a supplement to the public social security program for retirees. Some pensions have been established by individual private employers, others through collective bargaining agreements between trade unions and employers, and in a small number of cases individuals have established their own retirement pension plans. Financing arrangements vary considerably, with employers financing some plans, and insurance companies, professional financial management companies, and trade unions responsible for the financing of other plans.

The provisions of pension plans qualified by the Treasury Department are now governed by federal pension law which regulates participation, vesting of benefits, options for spouses and other beneficiaries, funding standards, portability, plan termination, fiduciary standards, reporting and disclosure requirements, pension limitations, and individual incentives (see Chapter 6).

"Nearly one-half of all workers in commerce and industry in the United States and three-fourths of all government civilian personnel are now enrolled in retirement plans other than OASDI (Social Security). . . . This number is estimated to be about 50 million" (Institute of Life Insurance, 1975). There is some evidence to indicate that the growth of private pension plans has been slowing in recent years and that it is unlikely that a greater percentage of the total labor force will have access to such plans in the future (Koludrubetz, 1975).

Often both long service and full retirement are required in order for pension benefits to be paid. At present these types of provisions are rarely modified to allow for a flexible retirement age. Basically, there are four types of retirement flexibility provisions in private pension plans: (1) pension always paid at a fixed age irrespective of employment; (2) pension paid at a fixed age with the provision that employment stops; (3) pension paid when employment stops; (4) pension paid when health problems or disability cause employment to stop; (or combinations of the above).

In the United States a large number of manufacturing and retail enterprises have established private pension plans. Tax reductions and collective bargaining between trade unions and private employers have contributed to the growth of these plans. Under the Employee Retirement Income Security Act of 1974 (ERISA), an employer must meet certain vesting requirements to assure that workers retain some portion of future pension benefits. As a result of these requirements, an employee must usually work a minimum of 10 to 15 years with the same employer to avoid loss of some pension rights. The common age to receive a full pension is generally the same as for Social Security benefits —age 65 for male workers and often age 60 or 62 for women. In some pension plans the retirement age is flexible between age 60 and 68. In some collectively bargained pension agreements, an employee may leave work with a full pension after 30 years service, irrespective of age. Pensions also are often somewhat higher between ages 60–65 in order to encourage early retirement before full Social Security benefits may be claimed. In general, although in theory many private pension plans allow persons to continue working beyond age 65, there is considerable encouragement to stop working when the regular pensionable age is reached.

Past Response of Older Workers to Retirement Choices.
Many variables enter into a worker's decision to retire, including retirement policies, expectations of income adequacy, health, and numerous personal desires. Whatever the reasons influencing individual decisions to retire, the pattern of response of older

workers to available retirement options has been very clear, especially since 1960. In that year 25 percent of currently payable, regular Social Security benefits to retired workers were reduced because of early retirement between ages 62 and 64. Since that time the percentage of persons retiring before 65 has increased dramatically: at present, more than half of new awards are reduced because of early retirement (Tables 3.2 and 3.3).

Reductions in the amount of benefits for persons who retire early are substantial. In 1974, when the average monthly regular Social Security payment was $193, the average for reduced awards was $162—a 17 percent reduction from the regular payment or about $360 per year less. The percentage of reduction in payments with early retirement has been increasing in recent years (Table 3). The trend toward early retirement in the United States is therefore very pronounced. More recent retirees have had favorable work and earnings histories and thus tend to receive greater Social Security payments at retirement. However the annual income received from these awards is still generally less than $4,000 per year, which certainly cannot be considered substantial in a period of significant cost increases (Fox, 1973).

The trend toward early retirement is probably encouraged by modifications in private pension plans that provide for a relatively low percentage of reduction in benefits with early retirement, and/or by supplemental early retirement payments until age 65, when full social security benefits can be claimed. In addition, workers with higher earning histories presumably may feel more financially able to retire since they will receive higher Social Security retirement benefits. Low-paid workers may feel that accepting reduced benefits while continuing to work (subject to the retirement test) may be most beneficial from a financial point of view. It remains for research to clarify further the multiple causes for early retirement decisions. What is clear, however, is that ever-increasing numbers of older workers are choosing to exercise early retirement options and that these decisions are having a significant effect on the age composition of the labor force.

Labor force participation rates for persons over 65 have been dropping steadily since 1960, when almost one of every three

Table 3.2 Numbers of Benefit Awards to Retired Workers with and without Reduction for Early Retirement, by Status of Award, 1956–1974

Year	Number(in thousands)					Reduced currently payable awards as percent of:		
	All awards	Currently payable regular[a]			Awards moving to payment status[b]	All awards	All currently payable regular awards[a]	All awards moving to payment status[b]
		Total	Not reduced	Reduced				
1956	934	890	775	115	909	12	13	13
1960	982	841	634	207	934	21	25	23
1961	1,362	1,166	629	537	1,284	39	46	42
1962	1,347	1,120	427	693	1,270	51	62	55
1963	1,146	964	351	613	1,066	54	64	58

1964	1,042	877	291	586	976	56	67	60
1965	1,183	875	296	579	979	49	66	59
1966	1,648	890	259	631	1,136	38	71	56
1967	1,161	763	127	636	1,032	55	83	62
1968	1,240	807	131	675	1,111	54	84	61
1969	1,273	808	119	689	1,141	54	85	60
1970	1,338	859	114	745	1,245	56	87	60
1971	1,391	919	120	799	1,259	57	87	63
1972	1,461	961	117	843	1,334	58	88	63
1973	1,493	1,047	135	912	1,548	61	87	60
1974	1,413	1,012	109	903	1,372	64	89	65

[a] Excludes disability conversions and transitionally insured as well as not currently payable awards.

[b] Currently payable regular awards plus estimate of those originally awarded as not currently payable that have moved to payment status; excludes conversions and awards to the transitionally insured.

Source: Social Security Administration (n.d.).

Table 3.3 Benefits (with Reduction for Early Retirement) Awarded and in Current-Payment Status for Individuals: Number and Average Monthly Amount After Reduction, by Age, 1974

Age	Awarded during year		In current-payment status at end of year	
	Number (in thousands)	Average monthly amount	Number (in thousands)	Average monthly amount
Total	1,020	$177.38	8,696	$169.50
62-64	759	165.10	1,631	158.60
62	459	152.82	438	152.50
63	187	175.24	568	158.10
64	113	198.33	646	163.40
65-69	261	213.03	3,439	177.50
65	243	215.82	813	179.80
66	19	176.56	762	179.80
67	–	–	673	176.40
68	–	–	613	176.00
69	–	–	578	174.20
70-74	–	–	2,256	170.20

70	—	526	—	173.50
71	—	490	—	171.60
72	—	456	—	169.90
73	—	399	—	168.80
74	—	385	—	166.00
75–79	—	1,128	—	163.50
75	—	317	—	165.80
76	—	299	—	165.30
77	—	250	—	164.60
78	—	154	—	159.00
79	—	109	—	155.40
80	—	95	—	153.30
81	—	81	—	151.90
82	—	62	—	148.50
83	—	3	—	147.00

Source: Social Security Administration (n.d.).

males over 65 was a full-time worker. In 1973 only about 20 percent of males over 65 were in the labor force. Projections indicate that this low rate is likely to continue through the year 2000. Shrinking labor force participation rates for older persons imply that the labor market is not readily accessible to them and that their contribution to national productivity is limited. Unfortunately, continuing high unemployment rates aggravate the difficulties normally encountered by older persons in trying to secure employment. In addition, although espousing full employment as a national policy objective, some major trade unions have recommended retirement as early as age 60 under the Social Security program while continuing to negotiate collectively with corporations for pension plan provisions permitting earlier and earlier retirement (AFL-CIO Executive Council, 1974). Private pension plans also have continued to provide incentives for early retirement. Therefore both public and private pension policies and the policies of trade unions appear to be designed to encourage early retirement, in some cases through the provision of positive incentives to leave full-time work. The response of the older population to current pension plan provisions has been *to utilize* early retirement options.

ECONOMIC CONSTRAINTS ON RETIREMENT PRACTICES

Historically there have been two basic points of view about when retirement should begin. One suggests that working beyond the "normal" retirement age may be psychologically and socially beneficial and may help maintain the proportionate size of the labor force. The other suggests that earlier retirement allows the individual the opportunity to enjoy extended leisure, opens positions of responsibility to younger persons, and facilitates reductions in the labor force made necessary by increasing automation. Neither of these points of view emphasizes the varying needs and preferences of older individuals or advocates a flexible approach to retirement. A flexible approach would include, at a minimum, the opportunity to leave the labor force at some time other than "normal" retirement age, to work less than the standard number of hours, or to change occupation.

It has been argued that if the conventional retirement age were increased, there would be little effect on retaining older persons (aged 65–69) within the labor force since many are already retired and no effect (except for changing the expectations) on persons aged 60–64, whereas if the retirement age were reduced, many persons in the 60–64 age group would move out of the labor force (Saville, 1963). This reasoning appears to accept the conventional ideas that older persons do not have the desire and capacity to work and that persons wish to leave full-time work at the earliest possible moment. When most of the incentives are designed to make earlier retirement more and more a possibility, it is not surprising that such a pattern of choice by older workers exists.

Although economic conditions are improving, the U.S. economy could continue to endure long-range unemployment at levels exceeding five percent. Irrespective of retired persons who may be seeking employment, it appears that there will be a continuing oversupply of labor in the future. Oversupply will persist because of the continuing automation of labor-intensive employment, and because of increases in the population needing employment. Thus automation will continue to reduce demand for workers, while population growth will provide a more than ample supply of workers.

The relatively high levels of unemployment which are likely to characterize the economy in the future will undoubtedly exert continuing pressure on older workers to retire and to accept a substantial loss in income. Thus a "flexible" early retirement policy will seemingly be forced upon many older workers. These workers will *sometimes* be replaced either by formerly unemployed persons or by members of the labor force who will maintain the national product, yet be responsible for increased transfer payments for the pensions of retired persons. If a national policy were established to greatly increase the relatively low incomes of the retired, there might be an increase in the overall propensity to consume both nondurable goods and services. This would probably gradually result in increased employment. However the effort needed to maintain such large transfer payments might well retard economic growth and be detrimental to the general economy.

We know that retirees suffer large losses in income when they leave regular full-time employment and subsequently do not share proportionately in overall improvements in the economy. Policies which provide incentives for early retirement frequently result in an increase in the magnitude of income loss for the retired worker and place the retiree at an even greater economic disadvantage. Certainly this economic disadvantage seems inequitable. Although a significant increase in retiree pensions through transfers is possible, such a policy would be extremely costly and would tend to raise serious financial problems which would likely limit economic growth (Saville, 1963). Current policies and resulting retirement trends are both economically and socially detrimental to older persons. They have few options to retire flexibly and it does not seem reasonable to expect older workers to continue to shoulder the burdens of automation and growth of the employable population.

Need for Retirement Flexibility.   A more general solution to these types of problems is necessary. Such a solution would certainly involve substantial new national policies directed toward providing more employment *in varying forms* and *for varying time periods* to those desiring work. A fundamental component of such a framework would be a public policy emphasizing retirement flexibility which would allow older workers much greater individual choice in dealing with the transition to retirement. Some of the options mentioned earlier, such as gradual retirement and re-employment subsequent to retirement would be important parts of a flexible retirement policy. Although governmental policy can be directed at increasing or decreasing the propensity to retire so as to adjust the size of the labor force, such an approach will not solve the basic problems of maintaining adequate economic growth with high levels of employment while accommodating both individual and social needs. A flexible retirement policy is not something which will solve fundamental economic problems. It is rather a means whereby an economy can increase the national product, decrease somewhat the burden of transfer payments, and provide opportunities for individuals to satisfy their own personal, social, and economic objectives in an environment relatively free from constraints on individuals.

Obstacles to Flexibility. There are a number of significant obstacles which frequently prevent older workers from retaining their jobs or securing new employment (Evans, 1973b). One obstacle is discrimination by employers against older workers. It is essential that deliberate discrimination in employment on the basis of age be eliminated as much as possible. Legislation prohibiting such discrimination (in the 45–65 age range) has been enacted in the United States. However such discrimination often takes place through the personnel policies of individual employers who fear declining work capacity and adaptability of older workers and utilize institutional policies and insurance rules to encourage or force older workers to retire. It is necessary to persuade employers to treat older workers equitably and to modify policies and insurance rules which discourage the employment of older workers. Such persuasion can realistically occur only through private business organizations and through governmental efforts to enforce broadened antidiscrimination legislation.

It has been observed that periods of high unemployment tend to affect older workers and that once they lose their jobs it is extremely difficult for them to find new ones. Because high unemployment is continuing, it is important that steps be taken to assist older workers who are particularly vulnerable to losing their jobs. Two particularly helpful approaches to this problem would be (1) specially designed job retraining courses for unemployed older workers; and (2) actions by federal and state employment services to discourage employers from imposing age limits in hiring and to provide special job transfer, job redesign, and job development programs for older workers.

A third serious problem which hinders the mobility and employability of older workers results from provisions of private pension programs which vest benefits only after long years of service and do not provide for transferability (portability) of pension benefits between employers. The Employee Retirement Income Security Act of 1974 protects the pension rights of workers through the establishment of vesting standards but does not encourage *very early* vesting or provide encouragement for transferability of pension rights. With the exception of a few industry-wide pension programs (such as the automobile industry), the principle of transferability of private pension rights has not been adopted in the United States. Therefore older workers feel that they cannot leave their present employers because they will jeopardize receipt of *full pension benefits* and because they are unsure of receiving a pension benefit from a proposed new employer. Thus both mobility and employability are being constrained by current pension plan practices.

When combined with current optional early retirement under the Social Security program, these incentives to retire become very difficult to resist. The problem of pension plan provisions that hinder employment of older workers is not easy to resolve, because underlying the current provisions is a set of society-wide beliefs about "appropriate time for retirement" and "making room for younger workers" which continue to condition the development of policy alternatives in the retirement field. Although certain modifications in public and private pension plans might be made to allow for greater flexibility for older workers, such incremental steps are likely to provide additional options only for selected groups of workers and to result in few incentives, so that current trends will not change. If greater flexibility is desired, a different set of beliefs and values concerning the need for and appropriateness of various work options for older people will have to be adopted by the government, private business, and trade unions.

RECOMMENDATIONS FOR CHANGE

Desirable Adjustments. Summarizing the issue of flexible retirement, we can say that many people wish to be able to cease work before reaching the regularly institutionalized retirement age. Others may want to continue working beyond the normal retirement age. In addition, there are some people who desire to work somewhat less than full-time and at less difficult kinds of jobs as they approach retirement. Adjustments which might be made to accommodate these desires include (1) changing regulations which require retirement at prescribed ages; (2) allowing persons to take time off during preretirement periods without mandating that they retire; (3) providing opportunities to transfer to less demanding jobs; and (4) providing opportunities for part-time work as employees age during both pre- and post-retirement periods. These changes might or might not be considered along with a general lowering or raising of the regular age of pension entitlement.

Solving the Income Problem. The main difficulty with the general adoption of the above recommendations lies in finding ways to provide income for individuals choosing various flexible retirement options. Solving the income problem would require changing many public and private pension program regulations to accommodate various forms of partial or temporary retirement. At present there are no provisions allowing persons to take a "temporary retirement" for one to two years while drawing an advance on their pension, then later returning to work. This might be approached by requiring a reduction in the level of pension benefit or by postponing final retirement beyond the regular retirement age. Also, there is now no provision that enables persons to work part-time and draw partial pension benefits, either before or after regular retirement.

The Need for Incentives. The cost of maintaining a large retired population is already substantial and is likely to rise even higher because of an increasing number of older persons, most of whom "choose" early retirement. In addition, higher levels of financial support are expected by retirees, and inflation continues to require cost-of-living raises in benefits to the retired population.

As pointed out, current policies provide few real incentives to continue work beyond the earliest possible age at which retirement benefits are granted. New approaches for flexible retirement certainly should provide incentives for older persons to remain at work if they wish to do so. Payment of partial retirement benefits to older persons who continue to work or significantly increasing final retirement benefits for those who postpone retirement might provide sufficient incentives for potential retirees to remain in the labor force while reducing the overall cost of pension benefits. Aside from purely economic considerations, the general well-being and morale of older persons would be improved by the knowledge that full retirement at a reasonable economic standard can be guaranteed from a certain age and that there is a viable option to continue employment and possibly to improve final income at retirement (Evans, 1973a).

Proposals for Income Transfers and Sabbaticals. There have been a number of recommendations for substantial policy changes to allow for greater flexibility in the work life. Although these types of change do not appear to lend themselves to development on an incremental basis, they represent new directions in thinking which should not be overlooked.

REHN PROPOSAL. One such recommendation calls for the creation of an integrated insurance system for transferring income between different periods of life (Rehn, 1973). This would mean combining many separate current programs for maintenance of income during periods of voluntary and involuntary nonemployment. The unified system would allow for individualized accounting, in which each person would be given the right to draw on his or her account for various purposes, including periods of leisure and education. Some limitations on drawing rights would have to be established to prevent accounts from being drawn down so far that sufficient funds for minimum old age pensions were endangered. In theory an individual could arrange to build up or deplete drawing rights at various times in his life in order to better satisfy individual preferences for work, leisure, and education.

Rehn believes that the introduction of an integrated income maintenance and transfer system would promote voluntary variations in the supply of labor without variations in individual income and would replace involuntary unemployment with education, retraining, or leisure. Moreover, the Rehn proposal introduces a new concept in social policy whereby incentives are offered to individuals to use their "own" funds to readjust within the labor market instead of waiting for the unemployment cycle to reach its peak. This type of more flexible transfer system points toward new approaches to the inflation-unemployment dilemma which has characterized our economy in recent years.

SUGARMAN PROPOSAL. A second and somewhat different type of flexible worklife proposal emphasizes periodic sabbatical leaves from employment with maintenance of income (Sugarman, 1975). This idea is based on the beliefs that full employment may not be an achievable goal and that the possibility of shared employment needs examination, research, and experimentation. Basically, the proposal known as the *decennial sabbatical plan* calls for a portion of individual earnings to be set aside for nine years; in every tenth year the sum accumulated would be sufficient to finance a year of income without employment. Individuals would be required to leave employment for one year out of each ten years, or to lose as much as 50 percent of their accumulated funds. Estimates suggest that about 70 percent of all salaried workers in the country would participate in the plan and that a large capital fund would quickly be accumulated which would be available to the government or private firms to meet investment needs. The major objective of the proposal is to make it possible to divide employment more equitably among those who wish to participate in the labor force.

CHANGING PERSPECTIVES ON WORK, LEISURE, AND EDUCATION

The study of New Patterns for Working Time can be regarded as an investigation of the impact of a new technology upon values. That is, a flexible work schedule or a shorter work week, as it becomes a more typical pattern, assumes the status of a technological development. As with any major technological change, alterations may be expected in value systems. These altered values, in turn, will be reflected in labour laws and contracts, family life, trade union philosophy and tactics, political orientations, employment stability and mobility, economic theory, educational philosophy and other aspects of the social system (Glickman, 1973, p. 141).

In the past, considerable attention has been focused on the numerous economic, sociological, and psychological aspects of work. More recently, the time spent by individuals in paid employment has gradually declined, and this trend is likely to continue in the years ahead. With this decrease in working time has come an increased amount of nonwork time which is devoted to leisure, rest, and education. New patterns of time utilization are developing and new perspectives and criteria are needed to study changing patterns of work, leisure, and education. It is important to recognize that work and leisure are combined in the individual's lifespace and are not separate and clearly divisible parts of human behavior.

Over the next 25 years we can expect some significant changes in the emphasis on work-centered and leisure-centered values. It is quite likely that significant experimentation with new patterns of work and leisure will take place during this period, despite limited information regarding the feasibility of various proposals for change. The general direction of future change is toward greater flexibility in work and leisure patterns. In considering future change, it is important to examine flexible alternatives in terms of given conditions at different points in time. From a policy viewpoint, the issue is one of establishing directions for change that reflect basic objectives and are feasible in terms of the economic, demographic, and social conditions at particular times.

Individual choice can operate only within limits established by structural and regulatory constraints. Restrictions on individual action are imposed and the options to be allowed are established by law, contracts, and collective bargaining. Government is continually involved in adjusting economic policy, incorporating policy choices which determine the ranges of choice available to employers and employees. Therefore to effect fundamental change it is necessary to make *work life flexibility* a specific and expressed goal of public policy and to establish some organizational structure which would be responsible for achieving this goal. It certainly is possible that an active government policy committed to more flexible employment could help to regularize production and employment and provide greater potential for adjustment to moderate growth or decline of job availability (Evans 1973b; Glickman, 1973).

Government should also assume a leadership role in supporting the research needed to understand better how individuals currently view the distribution of their time between employment and leisure, how such views change over time, what new options might be preferred and utilized, and how individuals could be best prepared to adjust to upcoming changes in time allocation. In conducting various types of research, many long-accepted values and beliefs must be reviewed as the frame of reference shifts from concern with conditions of employment to a much broader perspective involving the distribution of time in general. Many additional variables will have to be introduced into the analysis, and thus problem definition, analysis, and policy formulation will become somewhat more difficult.

> Certainly the choices are not clear cut. How much individual autonomy can the social and economic system accept? There are undoubtedly limits that the system can assimilate and tolerate with regard to flexibility of schedules, diversity of values and life styles and independent functioning in a self-actualizing mode. Such questions as these require that the structural and psychological characteristics affecting choices across a whole range of rigid and flexible systems be better understood. . . . Until basic policy choices are made and the socio-economic system becomes re-stabilized in whatever new basic modes come to prevail, it is possible that many innovations with worthwhile potential may be discarded because they are evaluated in narrow perspectives against short term criteria and not in terms of the longer term model of broad scope (Glickman, 1973, pp. 163, 165).

A great deal of further experimentation and research is necessary; after such experimentation is completed, the implementation of effective approaches and alternatives should naturally follow. Certainly, a more leisure-oriented society cannot come into existence without more training and education for the constructive use of leisure. New patterns for the utilization of time must be functionally and structurally integrated into the social fabric of the society so that a higher quality of life with more freedom of choice for each individual is achieved.

REFERENCES

AFL-CIO Executive Council. *Lowering the retirement age.* Washington, D.C.: AFL-CIO, 1974.

Ball, R. M. Social security financing. *Public Welfare,* 1975, *33*(4), 10–16.

Barkin, S. Pension systems and continued employment for the aged. In *Flexibility of retirement age.* Paris: Organization for Economic Cooperation and Development, 1970.

de Chalendar, J. (Ed.). *New patterns for working time.* Paris: Organization for Economic Cooperation and Development, 1973.

The elderly in America. *Population Bulletin,* 1975, *30,* 3–5.

Evans, A. A. Life-long distribution of working time. In J. de Chalendar, (Ed.), *New patterns for working time, supplement to the final report.* Paris: Organization for Economic Cooperation and Development, 1973a.

Evans, A. A. *Flexibility in working life.* Paris: Organization for Economic Cooperation and Development, 1973b.

Fox, A. Income of newly entitled beneficiaries 1970. *Survey of newly entitled beneficiaries* (Report No. 10). Washington, D.C.: U.S. Department of Health, Education and Welfare, Social Security Administration, June 1973.

The Growth of Output. Paris: Organization for Economic Cooperation and Development, 1970.

Glickman, A. S. Policy problems. In J. de Chalendar. (Ed.), *New patterns for working time, supplement to the final report.* Paris: Organization for Economic Cooperation and Development, 1973.

Hyden, S. Flexible retirement provisions in public pension systems. In *Flexibility of retirement age.* Paris: Organization for Economic Cooperation and Development, 1970.

Institute of Life Insurance. *Pension facts of 1975.* New York: Institute of Life Insurance, 1975.

Kahn, H., & Weiner, A. J. *The year 2000: A framework for speculation on the next thirty-three years.* New York: Macmillan, 1967.

Kolodrubetz, W. Employee benefit plans, 1973. *Social Security Bulletin,* 1975, *38*(5), 22–29.

Kreps, J. *Lifetime allocation of work and leisure* (Research Report No. 22). Washington, D.C.: U.S. Department of Health, Education and Welfare, Social Security Administration, Office of Research and Statistics, 1968.

Maric, D. Picture, country by country and branch by branch of the actual duration of time worked. In J. de Chalendar. (Ed.), *New patterns for working time, supplement to the final report.* Paris: Organization for Economic Cooperation and Development, 1973.

Moore, G. H., & Hedges, J. N. Trends in labor and leisure. *Monthly Labor Review,* 1971, *94*(2), 3–11.

Morrison, M. H. The myth of employee planning for retirement. *Industrial Gerontology,* 1975, *2*(2), 135–143.

Organization for Economic Cooperation and Development. *The growth of output.* Paris: OECD, 1970.

Pechman, J. A. *Making economic policy: The role of the economist.* General Series Reprint 311. Washington, D.C.: The Brookings Institution, 1976.

Rehn, G. Prospective view on patterns of working time. In J. de Chalender (Ed.), *New patterns for working time, supplement to the final report.* Paris: Organization for Economic Cooperation and Development, 1973.

Rustant, M. Economic development in the 1970's and its implications for employment. In J. de Chalendar. (Ed.) *New patterns for working time, supplement to the final report.* Paris: Organization for Economic Cooperation and Development, 1973.

Samuelson, P. A. *Newsweek,* November 16, 1970.

Saville, L. Flexible retirement. In J. Kreps (Ed.) *Employment income and retirement problems of the aged.* Durham, N.C.: Duke University Press, 1963.

Social Security Administration, Office of Research and Statistics, Unpublished data, no date.

Sugarman, J. M. Testimony of Jule M. Sugarman, Chief Administrative Officer, City of Atlanta, U.S. Congress, Joint Economic Committee, December 8, 1975 (mimeo).

Retirement Age Policies and Options for Employment in Europe

R. Meredith Belbin

Retirement poses two distinct types of problem. There is the problem posed for society (and two of its constituent entities, the firm and the pension fund) by the creation of another dependent, and there is the problem posed for the individual who finds himself threatened with loss of function, role, status, and perhaps economic security, for even the security which people believe they enjoy often contains an element of doubt. A well-known British comedian, Eric Morecambe, expressed the point rather sharply when interviewed about his retirement plans: "Show business people are never as rich as others think they are. But personally I've got enough money to last me for the rest of my life. Provided I die at 6 o'clock tonight." When longevity, inflation, and early retirement coincide, insolvency may be just around the corner.

Clearly there is a limited number of possibilities for combining employment and retirement in systems that give heed to individual choice and at the same time remain economically viable. Both banks of the Atlantic—if in this era of advanced telecommunications we liken the Atlantic to a small river—must share similar problems, and so any system that is tested and adopted on one bank will probably prove equally good on the other. This may suggest, therefore, that what I have to say about the other bank is hardly likely to prove new and startling. After all, if the soil is similar on both banks the vegetation is likely to be similar also. Nevertheless, I will maintain that the differences in soil structure are large enough to support ecological variation, and this means that the seeds can blow across the Atlantic river, in either direction, and take root on the other side.

Before elaborating on this theme, I want to say a few words about the common climate of opinion on both banks, bearing in mind that it is only when the climate is suitable that seeds can germinate and plants can grow. The climate of the times has been set for us by two bodies, of which both the United States and European countries are fellow members. These bodies are the United Nations, and in particular its specialized agency, the International Labor Organization in Geneva, and the Organization for Economic Cooperation and Development in Paris. Over the years these organizations have had some important things to say.

In 1962 the International Labor Organization received at its 46th Session the report of its Director-General on "Older People: Work and Retirement." In a concluding section, David A. Morse wrote:

> Premature withdrawal from work is a burden on any community and an obstacle to economic and social advancement. As such it needs to be combated with unrelenting vigor. Ideally all people who wish to go on working and are capable of work should be able to find and retain suitable employment. If this goal is to be reached—and we are still far from it in most parts of the world—many-sided community efforts are needed to maintain full employment and to enable older people to adapt to structural changes in employment and to claim their fair share of employment opportunities. (International Labor Organization, 1975, p. 96).

In 1970 the General Assembly of the United Nations recommended that "a high priority be given to the question of the elderly." The Secretary General was asked to report on this to the Economic and Social Council in 1973 and to the General Assembly in 1974. In a preliminary note prepared in 1972, the Secretary General requested developed countries as well as developing countries to review the question of mandatory retirement. He urged consideration of "flexible retirement and income insurance, which would allow workers to choose their age of retirement according to income needs or other personal factors, or to switch to other work for which their skills, experience, and perhaps retraining might suit them without depriving younger men of job opportunities." In fact, in 1970 the Organization for Economic Cooperation and Development had already published a comprehensive report on "The Flexibility of Retirement Age" (Barkin, 1970). In 1971 OECD followed this up with publication of a policy document which included the following declaration:

> The Manpower and Social Affairs Committee believes that increased possibilities for individual choice should be available as between leisure and work, particularly for mature and older workers. Flexibility in this sense would also be in line with changes as to working capacity and energy associated with ageing and yet give recognition to the fact that older people are usually reluctant to make drastic changes in the style of life to which they have grown accustomed. . . .
>
> The Manpower and Social Affairs Committee recognises that the widening of choice may lead a significant proportion of workers to opt either for continued employment over the traditional retiring age or for an intermediate condition of partial retirement and part-time employment or for early retirement (definitive or temporary) with the appropriate actuarial consequences. At present, it is not possible to do more than speculate on how individuals would react to this increased freedom of choice. . . .
>
> The Manpower and Social Affairs Committee believes that if a higher participation rate of middle-aged and older workers can be combined with increased individual choice to enter or leave the labour market, there could be real benefits for all age groups of society. . . .
>
> The Manpower and Social Affairs Committee, therefore, proposes that Member countries should give consideration to ways of establishing the facts about individuals' behaviour over a period of time when retirement options are presented. Such fact-finding exercises might take the form of localised experiments where these are feasible within the existing social security system or a follow-up of individuals who already have an option under existing schemes (Organization for Economic Cooperation and Development, 1971, p. 7).

The most recent policy statement of a major international body comes from the 1975 report issued by the United Nations Department of Economic and Social Affairs entitled "The Aging: Trends and Policies." This report contains a number of vigorous declarations:

> A policy on aging is essential in order to assure the increasing numbers and proportions of older persons their basic human rights —full participation and contribution to, as well as protection in, the society of which they are a part.
>
> Social policies and programmes must recognize the resources to be found within a specific segment of the older population, such as levels of education, ability to work and voluntary capabilities, among others. In other words, policies must avoid the identification of only negative situations confronting older persons as defined by unmet needs. They must also recognize the positive attributes and potential contributions of older persons and provide for the development of programmes to assure productive roles for them.
>
> Long-term goals and policy development must include the right of older persons to work, as well as the right to choose retirement from work in old age. In many countries retirement is mandatory based upon chronological age and not on capacities and capabilities. . . . For countless individuals who are still in their middle years, age may become a factor in discriminatory practices, barring their entry or re-entry into the labour force (United Nations, 1975, pp. 51, 53, 55).

The report concludes with the recommendations of the expert group meeting on aging held at the United Nations headquarters during May 1974. These recommendations include two important points:

> The aging population has the right to share in the social, cultural and economic development of their nation. Society has the right and obligation to provide the means for the aging to continue to contribute to this development. . . .
>
> Governments should develop policies to prohibit discrimination in employment due to age (United Nations, 1975, pp. 69, 72).

To sum up, it seems that over the last decade there has been a certain consensus among experts that society needs to carry a lower burden of economically dependent older people, that older people still possess the potential to contribute to society, and that society should take advantage of this by finding the means to exercise this potential. In doing so, freedom of choice should be extended to offer the options of continuing work, retiring, and phasing out employment.

This consensus has been reinforced by the developing nature of research. We have now passed the era when our assessment of individual preferences concerning work and retirement hinged on simplistic questions about whether or not individuals wanted retirement. People adjust to the inevitable. We now realize that it is much more difficult to assess underlying aspirations which indicate how people would exercise their options if given a greater choice.

Nevertheless, we have some leads and these leads support the recommendations from the international bodies cited above. My own studies (Belbin & Clark, 1970) of retirement rates for different occupations in the United Kingdom and the studies of Jaffe (1970) in the United States independently reached very similar conclusions. People in self-employed occupations, including those with higher incomes, tend to retire late. In the United Kingdom the ratio of self-employed workers to retirees in the older age groups is higher among professional men than among any other group listed in the census. Jaffe found that late retirement is associated not only with higher life income but also with higher education. In general, where people control their own working arrangements, conditions, and time of retirement, the net effect seems to be that early retirement is more than counterbalanced by late retirement. Where that personal control is absent, as in large corporations, early retirement is much more pronounced than late retirement.

A study on the retirement preferences of 55–64-year-old workers in three United Kingdom firms (Jacobsohn, 1970) found that the initial attitude toward retirement shifted in a significant way once other possibilities presented themselves (Table 4.1). Whereas most workers tended to favor retirement over continuing at work, only one in five workers favored complete retirement once offered the option of working at a reduced level.

Such findings are in keeping with gerontological psychology, which suggests that as people age they become more resistant to sudden changes in their life styles. A phased reduction in work load is exactly what gerontological psychologists would prescribe.

Table 4.1 Attitude Towards Part-Time or Occasional Employment Among Retirement- and Work-Oriented Respondents

Preference as to form of employment by firm after pensionable age	All		Initial attitude towards retirement	
	N	%	Willing N=119	Reluctant N=96
Full-time employment	33	15.4	–	34.4
Regular part-time employment	84	39.1	34.5	45.0
Occasional employment	52	24.2	26.9	20.6
Complete withdrawal from work	46	21.3	38.6	–
	215	100.0%	100.0%	100.0%

Source: Jacobsohn (1970).

In the light of this and similar research evidence and of the authoritative pronouncements of international organizations quoted earlier, what has been the response of government? Governments should, one would suppose, have a real interest in promoting the rights of older people to participate in economic life, for a large dependent population imposes a heavy burden on the working population. In Europe this burden has been growing in a progressive and alarming fashion. If we take the latest rates of male activity in the labor force (published in the ILO Yearbook for 1975) and compare them with similar figures of 10 years ago, we find that male activity rates for all ages have fallen in all 20 European countries. The rate stood at 60 percent or more in 12 of 20 European countries in the early 1960s, but the 12 had shrunk to four by the early 1970s. Whereas only eight countries had rates as low as between 50 and 59 percent in the 1960s, by the early 1970s the figure doubled to 16. Overall, the last decade has seen a drop of male activity rates in Europe from about 61 percent to something nearing 56 percent.

In fact the response of European governments to this developing problem has been barely perceptible. Of course it is clear that as things stand at present, those two large pressure groups, business corporations and trade unions, have a minimal interest and sometimes even a counter-interest in promoting the cause of older workers by retaining them in, or adding them to, the labor force. Whenever organizations have run into temporary problems, government seems to have gone along with the tide in facilitating the laying off of older workers. The United Kingdom is typical of many European countries in having enacted "redundancy arrangements" whereby employers are obliged to compensate discharged workers according to length of service. Since "voluntary redundancy" is now the favored pattern for shedding manpower because of its acceptability to employees and trade unions, older workers are more tempted than younger workers to declare themselves for "redundancy." After collecting a large lump sum in cash, a high proportion then seek to regain their old jobs once demand recovers. But often demand fails to recover to its former level, or that level is achieved by higher productivity.

Older workers who have been forced or coaxed into premature retirement usually have great difficulty in finding alternative employment when they decide to seek it.

Pressures that enforce early retirement not only cause individual hardship but also, in a broader sense, threaten damage and shock to traditional cultures. Switzerland might offer a case in point. Here is a country in which small firms and family businesses thrive and in which older people readily find appropriate roles. The prosperity which Switzerland has enjoyed—well indicated by the strength of the Swiss franc—might offer, on economic grounds alone, a basis for the support of a large retirement population. But, paradoxically, as Table 4.2 shows, the latest statistics permitting international comparisons place Switzerland in the front rank of European countries for the industriousness of its older people. That pattern now at last seems to be changing not as a result of prosperity but as a consequence of world-wide recession. M. Villars of the Swiss Office Federale des Assurances Sociales has recently reported:

> Full employment has meant that every pensioner who wanted to work could find a paid job whether full or part time. Approximately 60% of retired people took up such work in the first few years of their pension. [In Switzerland the granting of an old age pension is not conditional on giving up all paid work.] . . . Until the recent worsening of the economic situation, the federal, cantoral and municipal authorities were hardly aware of . . . the problems of retirement.

The importance of culture may be inferred from Table 4.2, which illustrates the wide variation in European nations' pattern of response to the retirement years. Prosperity, size of country, and political complexion evidently have no important bearing on activity rates in later maturity. On a simple guess, it seems likely that the Swiss have continued to work because they are a hard-working people while their early-retiring neighbors, the Austrians, are happy-go-lucky. If culture acts as a major determinant of work and retirement patterns, then these patterns can clearly be disrupted, with socially damaging consequences, by economic forces that man has not as yet succeeded in controlling.

Table 4.2 European Male Activity Rates in Higher Age Groups

Country	Year	Age	
		60-64 %	65+ %
Austria	1971	44.9	8.0
Belgium	1970	63.8	6.8
Bulgaria	1965	55.1	23.0
Czechoslovakia	1970	33.3	14.6[a]
Denmark	1970	81.4	23.5
Faroe Isles	1970	84.1	35.4
Finland	1970	63.1	13.8
France	1968	65.7	19.3
Germany E.	1971	83.4	27.2
Germany W.	1970	69.4	16.1
Greece	1971	65.9	31.9
Holland	1971	74.8	13.1
Ireland	1971	87.6	43.9
Italy	1971	40.6	13.4
Leichtenstein	1970	85.8	41.8
Luxembourg	1970	45.5	10.1

Norway	1970	79.0	25.7
Poland	1970	83.0	56.4[a]
Portugal	1970	79.1	52.9
Rumania	1966	67.6	39.3[a]
Spain	1970	74.2	21.4
Switzerland	1970	87.3	31.7
Sweden	1970	75.7	15.2
UK	1971	86.5	19.3
Yugoslavia	1971	62.7	50.9[a]
Compare			
United States	1970	73.0	24.8
Japan	1970	85.8	54.4

[a]65–70 only.
Source: ILO Yearbook of Labor Statistics (1975).

The latest European statistics in Table 4.2 do not reflect the impact of the current recession, but it is already clear that the shedding of manpower has had a disproportionate effect on employment statistics in the upper age groups. Now the question is whether Europe, through the Council of Europe and the Commission of European Communities, will respond to this challenge.

The answer, I would submit, falls into three parts.

First, there is a growing awareness of the problem, but this awareness has not transformed itself into policy measures that are as radically comparable as those adopted in other fields. One of the reasons for this is the belief that the recession will be short-lived and that equilibrium will be re-established. If this fails to happen, a major policy response seems possible.

Second, a number of short-term measures have been taken that have already proved effective in averting hardships and major social problems in particular localities. In 1972 the Commission of the European Communities set up the New European Social Fund. Article Five of the Fund states that:

> Assistance shall be granted for measures for the absorption and reabsorption into active employment of the disabled, and of older workers, women, and young workers.

Provision is made for:

> Aid for eliminating obstacles which make it difficult for certain categories of disadvantaged workers to take up available employment. . . . This aid shall cover necessary expenses incurred in helping to maintain the level of earnings of elderly workers who undergo vocational retraining; this allowance, payable over a maximum period of six months, shall be granted in respect of workers of between 50 years of age and the legal age of obtaining an old-age pension.

In practice, money from this fund is being used to facilitate redeployment. For example, workers in the overmanned steel industry in South Wales have been invited to "volunteer for redundancy." Those who volunteer tend to be highly paid and have often had many years of service. Their redundancy (leaving) gratuity reflects earnings and length of service, and so on discharge they collect an appreciable sum of money. They then have an inducement to transfer into another, possibly poorly paid job outside the industry. The immediate level of earnings is not important because their income is in any case guaranteed at its former level for six months through money from the fund.

The third answer to the question we have posed must by its very nature be speculative, because it concerns policy options both in the immediate and the distant future. Yet there are grounds for making reasonable presumptions about the directions which these policy options will take.

In the first place it is unlikely that the European community will acquiesce in a continuing employment squeeze on those in the older age groups. Many countries in Europe are very conscious of their cultural traditions and way of life and are highly resistant to particular forms of employment disruption and consequential social disturbance that are associated with the personnel policies of large firms and multinational corporations in particular. The right to work is virtually acknowledged in Europe. In the view of many, that right must be made a reality. The delicate balance of political forces in Europe cannot allow it to be otherwise.

There is in any case less compunction in Europe, I believe, than in the United States about the role and responsibilities of government in intervening in social and economic affairs. That at least is the impression I have gained after shuttling to and fro between the United States and Europe a good number of times. Observing that this difference exists at all points along the political spectrum, left, right, and center, I have reflected on its underlying reasons. The mistrust which, as an onlooker, I witness among Americans toward their own federal government may have its roots in a conflict of responsibilities between federal government and state government. This mistrust is also a consequence in part, one supposes, of the immense size of the United States, the physical remoteness of most people from the seat of government, and the size of the bureaucracy which serves its needs. Perhaps it is not for me to comment on the internal affairs of the United States. The only reason for doing so is to draw attention to some basic contrasts in Europe. The European community contains some small but very influential nations. For example, half the population of Denmark lives in Copenhagen. The sense of intimacy between government and people is almost akin to that between citizens and town councils in some much larger countries. Government is obliged to be aware of the expectations which an active and local electorate places upon it and which involve all aspects of well-being.

Social and economic innovators have only small obstacles to overcome in small countries. Once policies have been applied, they readily lend themselves to dissemination through international organizations. Sweden, for example, has already made its mark on more than one occasion as a small country pioneer. The Active Manpower Policy which OECD recommended to member countries in the late 1950s had strong Swedish connections and proven experience behind it. In this era training was to become a centerpiece of labor policy. The Manpower Development Training Act in the United States and the Industrial Training Act in the United Kingdom were both enacted during this period, and although both acts were adapted to national needs, similar features testify to common origins.

It seems possible, therefore, that any one of a number of countries might alight on some new policy affecting work and retirement, and that favorable experience with that policy could recommend it for wider adoption. This seems more probable than the possibility that international organizations will conjure up radically new policies out of the blue, as it were, and persuade member countries to adopt them.

What then are the prospects of any major new developments in Europe?

Concern for the employment prospects of those in later maturity and for personal liberty in the timing of retirement has not of itself attracted any large body of support in any country. Older people are apt to accept the established social order and to struggle toward individual rather than collective resolution of their problems. However, it does seem that where issues concerning older workers are tied to allied issues, there are prospects of major changes ahead. Two options are already presenting themselves, one based on an extension of the right to work and the other as a consequence of a developing investment in lifelong education.

The United Kingdom provides an example of a possible development in the first direction. Because of the prevalence of juvenile rates of pay, youths in the United Kingdom have never experienced high unemployment. Over time, this difference between juvenile and adult rates of pay has been eroded, and there is now a greater prevalence of paying for the job rather than according to the age of the worker. At any rate the present recession has set off rising unemployment among the young, which, as it happens, has coincided with soaring juvenile crime. The government has responded on two fronts. Firms have in effect been paid to take on unemployed school-leavers, and, more significantly, guaranteed work has been provided in depressed areas. This work has been mainly organized through a body called Community Industry and funded by the Manpower Services Commission, which incidentally also oversees the Employment Services Agency and the Training Services Agency. What started as a local experiment has now turned into a national system which is growing rapidly.

Once established, institutions designed for a particular age group tend to extend their age range. In any case, institutions seem to operate more successfully when the age structure of their work populations are in balance. In Northern Ireland, Enterprise Ulster operates in a similar way to Community Industry, except that in providing both work and training it caters to the unemployed over the whole prepensionable age span. Enterprise Ulster has continued to make headway in spite of the difficulties occasioned by the grave security problems in Ulster.

What seems to be happening is that the "right to work" is already operating, not as yet in a comprehensive way, but on a local scale in selected areas. At least the institutions that serve this purpose are being built up. As the numbers of older entrants in these institutions grow, so will the knowledge and experience on how best to meet the needs of the prepensionable older worker.

The second significant move which may ultimately have a major bearing on work and retirement options in the higher age groups comes from France. France has always had a strong tradition of central government. Workers of any age in France now have a right established by law, though subject to a number of specific conditions, to take paid leave and to avail themselves of courses of further education and training, including preparation for retirement. French employers are obliged to contribute a one percent levy of their wage bill to the state to pay for the country's system of lifelong education (education permanente). This levy is shortly due to be doubled to two percent. It is interesting that the French Parliament has ruled that preretirement training falls within the definition of "vocational training as part of lifelong education."

One must remark that French moves have struck some of their European partners as somewhat extreme, but their severity may be mitigated if there is any truth in the allegation that French laws are not observed anyway! Nevertheless, the importance of these French moves should not be underestimated. The right to continuing education and training carries implications for the developing role of older people in society. Training, in particular, implies preparation. But preparation for what? Once expectations are fostered by involvement in further education and training, it is difficult to believe that a new breed of middle-aged, regenerated Frenchmen will be content to accept a "roleless role."

These two developments, based on the right to work and the right to further education and training, may be likened to starter-cultures. The fermentation may produce a rich brew at some time in the future. However it is anyone's guess as to how the brew will turn out. The present programs have not yet been adapted to take account of the specific needs and problems of older people in society. Here one has to admit that in Europe generally, with only occasional exceptions, there is much less sophisticated awareness of this subject than in the United States. The United States contributes a major share of the total world research in gerontology. And this effort is reflected in that pioneering approach which was expressed in these chapters.

With this spirit in mind we can at least consider the shape and forms which work and retirement *ought* to take in Europe, if Europe is to make any impact on this front. Here gerontological research has something relevant and important to say: that the most promising line of advance lies through a gradual and controlled phasing out from work. Since advocacy of both phasing out and flexible retirement has achieved nothing, as we have seen, over the last decade, the onus falls on government to set the scene or at least to lead the way. How can this be done?

Michael Fogarty, whose recent (1976) book on middle age has caused a considerable stir, recently convened a seminar on the Future of Pensions at the Centre for Studies in Social Policy in London. His paper contained the following statement:

> A policy permitting substantial savings could be to provide that all pensions—social security or occupational, and whether actuarially reduced for early retirement or not—should be paid at half-rate until, say, age 70, except in the case of disablement. The assumption would be that young and able pensioners could and should normally seek at least part-time work. A condition would of course be the final abolition of the earnings rule, and action to ensure that opportunities for appropriate work were actually available (p. 145).

The idea of paying a part-pension is an interesting one. The drawback is that firms are reluctant to employ part-timers. Additional backup measures are clearly needed. Both the carrot and the stick can be considered. The carrot might take the form of tax relief or relief from Social Security payments for employees over the age of 55 who are engaged in part-time employment. The stick one shrinks to recommend. Nevertheless, a seemingly harsh measure would open wide the road to progress if the firing of employees when they reached a fixed age were to count as illegal age discrimination. In place of fixed age retirement, progressive retirement would be permissible from the age at which employees first became eligible for a part-pension. The scene would then be set for managers to turn their attention to the most effective way of using the contributions of which older employees are capable.

The notion of work-sharing, inherent in the idea of graduated retirement, might also offer the basis for a fruitful dialogue with the trade unions. (In Europe unions have often favored work-sharing in preference to the discharge of union members.)

Compatible with the suggestion of a statutory basis to graduated retirement is an idea first developed by Brandon at a seminar on the Older Worker held in London in 1974 under the auspices of the Industrial Society. Brandon proposed a personnel policy for executives which would extend compulsory retirement until 70, subject to certain provisions. These were that after the age of 40 no executive would be allowed to occupy the same post or level for more than four years. He would then either be promoted or demoted with compensation from a special fund or offered part-time work and a part-time pension. According to Brandon's calculations such a system would increase the promotion prospects of talented younger men, offer the retention in service of talented older executives, and open up a normal procedure for redeploying others in work suitable to their abilities and energies. The prospect of drawing an early part-pension would make Brandon's plan even more workable.

Progress in monitoring and pursuing the various options, in developing new experimental programs, and in disseminating what is known and effective requires resources. In Europe the funding of research in aging has fallen a long way behind the standard set in the United States. Without adequate funding it is difficult to believe that any major programs will have the rocket boost needed for them to get into orbit. Some part of these much-needed resources might well be derived from pension funds. At the London meeting at which Fogarty presented his paper, it was proposed that one percent of pension funds might usefully be earmarked for research. Vast sums of money are now locked up in pension funds. The way in which that money is ultimately used is a matter of major importance. A wise use of accrued benefits might do much to improve the lot and happiness of that massive population that stands on the verge of retirement and can still consider its options.

To finish as I began, one cannot but be impressed by the similarity of the problems of aging on both sides of the Atlantic. Human experience is the most communicable of all subjects.

What goes on in the United States in the field of aging cannot and will not be ignored in Europe. Europe in its turn may one day stumble on some formula or approach which may also merit attention in the U.S. But by confering with American experts about our mutual experiences, we may stumble less.

REFERENCES

Barkin, S., et al. *Flexibility of retirement age.* Paris: Organization for Economic Cooperation and Development, 1970.

Belbin, R. M., & Clark, F. G. Relationship between retirement pattern and work. *Industrial Gerontology,* 1970, *4,* 12–26.

Belbin, R. M., & Belbin, E. *Problems in adult retraining.* London: Heinemann, 1972.

Belbin, R. M., & Belbin, E. Retraining and the older worker. In D. Pym (Ed.), *Industrial society: Social science in management.* London: Penguin, 1969.

The discovery method: An international experiment in retraining. *Employment of older workers 6.* Paris: Organization for Economic Cooperation and Development, 1969.

Fogarty, M. P. *Pensions—where next?* London: Centre for Studies in Social Policy, 1976.

International Labor Organization. *Older people: Work and retirement.* Report of the Director-General, Part I. Geneva: International Labor Office, 1962.

International Labor Office. *Yearbook of labor statistics.* Geneva: International Labor Office, 1975.

Jacobsohn, D. *Attitudes towards work and retirement among older industrial workers in three firms.* Unpublished doctoral thesis, London School of Economics and Political Science, 1970.

Jaffe, A. J. Men prefer not to retire. *Industrial Gerontology,* 1970, *5,* 1–11.

Organization for Economic Cooperation and Development. *Adaptation and employment of special groups of manpower: Implementing an active manpower policy.* Paris: Organization for Economic Cooperation and Development, 1971.

United Nations Department of Economic and Social Affairs. *The aging: Trends and policies.* New York: United Nations, 1975.

-Part III-

SOCIAL SECURITY AND PENSIONS

A multitude of public policy issues surrounds the public and private pension systems, and much analysis has been devoted to each. At this juncture, one key question—under which are subsumed many other important questions—emerges: What should be the relative future roles of Social Security and private pensions?

The issues are troublesome. Will continued emphasis on building up Social Security and increasing its benefits lead to the "crowding out" of private pension plans? Some businessmen, such as the Chairman of Sears Roebuck, are warning of just that eventuality. If this were to happen, Social Security benefits and taxes in the second quarter of the next century would need to be proportionately higher, and the burden of support for the elderly population bulge after 2010 would fall more heavily on future rather than present workers. In addition, some experts believe that reduced emphasis on private pensions would entail a reduction in funds available for investment, thus exacerbating a possible future shortage of capital.

On the other hand, de-emphasis of Social Security and increased reliance on private pensions would not be without costs and risks. Critics of employer and union pensions have long cited disadvantages such as their relatively high administrative costs; their susceptibility to willful or inadvertent mismanagement; inadequate vesting provisions leading to a loss of rights with job changes; the possibility that the availability of private pensions to better paid employees will reduce pressure to maintain adequate Social Security benefits for all; and the uncertain impact of pension fund investment upon the nation's economy.

These are problems we have tolerated for a long time. However, new and more substantial worries are now beginning to arise. If inflation persists or longevity increases, will plans be able to meet their promises? Will unfunded liabilities eventually prompt many terminations, leaving huge yearly insurance bills for taxpayers? How wise are the investment decisions being made by pension fund investors? Will the "prudent man" criteria set up by the 1974 pension reform result in overcautious investment decisions and the shunning of growth opportunities, with a resultant adverse effect on the economy as a whole?

In the chapters which follow, Alicia H. Munnell and Francis P. King address some of these issues and urge an expansion in the role of private pensions. Munnell would also like to see the present Social Security system altered substantially. The time has come, she says, to change Social Security into a pure retirement insurance program, turning over its other function—redistribution of income—to the Supplemental Security Income (SSI) program. SSI would then provide minimum benefits regardless of previous earnings and contributions to the system; Social Security would provide benefits in strict proportion to previous contributions; and private pensions (along with individual savings) would provide additional income for some workers. The projected shortfall in payroll revenues would be eliminated by shifting many people now receiving minimum Social Security benefits over to the SSI program, and then funding SSI solely through general revenues. Social Security would thus be divested of its welfare function and would become a pure retirement insurance plan.

Munnell argues that her proposal has several advantages. Needs-related subsidies would be paid from general revenues rather than the more regressive payroll tax. Overall costs would be lowered by preventing people who have worked only the minimum number of quarters but who have a second pension from receiving subsidized minimum Social Security benefits. Additionally, there would be less interference with private saving and more contribution to capital formation.

In his article on private and public employee pensions, Francis King makes two predictions: Congress is not likely to raise Social Security benefits further; and pension and profit-sharing plans will probably assume a greater role as future providers of retirement income. Questioning whether we can afford extensive early retirement provisions, King suggests that we may have to reexamine the present retirement age as well as the practice of mandatory retirement. Among the reforms he advocates are funding standards for state and municipal retirement systems, as well as earlier vesting requirements for all pension plans, public and private. He also urges that steps be taken to provide pension coverage for workers whose employers currently do not sponsor pension plans.

Both authors offer a provocative critique of current policies, but neither tackles the practical feasibility of their proposals or the controversial issues raised by them. King does not examine the impact on the economy or the administrative costs of his suggestions for expanding the private pension system. Munnell does not deal with the drawback that her proposal would require the transfer of many millions of workers to SSI, which is basically a welfare program and for many people bears a welfare stigma. The concluding chapter of this book discusses some of the issues raised by the two authors' proposals.

-5-

Social Security in a Changing Environment

Alicia Haydock Munnell

Social Security is a wonderful plan. People say it's going bankrupt. Don't believe them. It works. I know. My uncle reached 65 and he sent in the appropriate forms. In a week he received a wonderful letter: "Dear Mr. Gold, Welcome to the Social Security System. Attached is a list of 10 names. Just send $100 to each name on the list and type up a new list with your name at the bottom. But remember, don't break the chain!"

> Bobby Gold, *Parade Magazine* (March 28, 1976).

Today Social Security is an enormous program covering over 90 percent of the working population and dispensing $83 billion annually in benefits to the retired, the disabled, and their dependents and survivors. Current members of the system, working and retired, have been promised future benefits exceeding $4 trillion.

The growth of the Social Security program over the last 10 years has been unprecedented. Between 1966 and 1976, total benefit payments have ballooned from $20 billion to over $83 billion—a fourfold increase. Even after adjustment for inflation, benefits have doubled in the last decade. During the last five years real benefits rose at a rate of 50 percent between 1971 and 1976 when real Gross National Product (GNP) rose only 13 percent.

To finance this rapid expansion in benefits, Social Security taxes have also been significantly increased. In 1965, employers and employees paid a combined tax of 7.25 percent on the first $4,800 of wages; by 1975 the combined tax had increased to 11.7 percent of the first $14,100. In 1977 the maximum taxable wage base was increased again automatically to $16,500, so that the maximum tax levied on a covered worker has climbed from $348 to $1,930—more than a fivefold increase in the 12-year period.

Recently, the Social Security system has come under considerable criticism as its opponents question its long-run financial viability in the face of dramatic demographic shifts coupled with the potential imbalance caused by the present overindexed benefit formula, which overcompensates future retirees for cost of living increases.* The large forecasted deficits are a legitimate cause for concern, and without modifications of the existing program, Social Security would require extraordinarily high tax rates after the turn of the century. Futhermore, if Social Security is to be successful, the program must adapt to a changing economic, social, and institutional environment.

This chapter discusses some of the recent developments and their implications for the future of Social Security. Primary emphasis will be on the old-age and survivors portion (OASI) of the old-age, survivors, disability, and health insurance (OASDHI) program; little attention will be given to the disability program, and health insurance is omitted entirely. Table I demonstrates the relative size and importance of OASI compared to the health and disability portions of the program.

THE ROLE OF SOCIAL SECURITY

The dimensions of Social Security will be shaped by two recent developments. The enactment in 1972 of the Supplemental Security Income (SSI) program, which provides federally established needs-related benefits to low-income elderly, preempts

---

*As this book was in press, Social Security legislation correcting this technical flaw was signed into law by President Carter (December 20, 1977).

Table I

DISTRIBUTION OF OASDHI BENEFITS BY

PROGRAM AND CLASS OF BENEFICIARY,

1975

Program and Type of Beneficiary	Benefits (billions)	Percentage of Total Benefits
Old-age and Survivors Insurance	$58.5	74.8
Retired workers	38.1	48.7
Dependents & Survivors	20.4	26.1
Persons with special age-72 benefits	.2	.2
Disability Insurance	8.4	10.7
Health Insurance	11.3	14.5
	78.2	100.0

Source: U.S. Department of Health, Education and Welfare, Social Security Administration, Office of Research and Statistics, unpublished data.
Note: Numbers may not add to totals due to rounding.

the welfare function of Social Security. At the other end of the income scale, the existence of the private pension system and recent evidence of the negative impact of Social Security on private saving place an upper limit on the desirable level of benefits. As discussed below, Social Security can now fulfill a unique role in a three-tiered retirement system—bounded at the bottom by SSI and at the top by the funded private pensions and individual saving so necessary for capital accumulation.

Supplemental Security Income Program.   Traditionally, Social Security has combined the goals of individual equity and social adequacy. Since 1939, the simple wage replacement role of Social Security has been supplemented by welfare functions such as a minimum benefit, dependents' benefits, and a steeply progressive benefit formula. This stress on social adequacy is appropriate in a social insurance program as long as the program is required to provide the major portion of retirement income.

Prior to 1974, most states provided for the needy aged, disabled, and blind through their federally supported public assistance programs. Each state set its own benefit levels and eligibility requirements. As a result, there were wide variations among states in the amount of support provided to these groups. Because state public assistance programs were largely independent of Federal policy, their existence did not serve to lessen the perceived burden of the income adequacy principle on Social Security. In fact, the growth of Social Security held down the number of old-age assistance recipients, because Social Security provided enough income to raise its beneficiaries above the need threshold.

Today, however, the welfare system has been significantly strengthened by the enactment in 1972 of the Supplemental Security Income (SSI) Program which replaces the old network of state systems with a single, federally financed and operated program of cash payments to the elderly, blind, and disabled. Under SSI, which is administered by the Social Security Administration and fully financed from general revenues, benefit levels, eligibility conditions, and means tests are uniform nationwide. States have the option of supplementing SSI payments, and are required to do so for those current recipients who would receive less under SSI than under the former Federal-state-local system.

Since SSI is a welfare program, applicants must prove need by conforming to certain income and asset limitations. As of July 1977, recipients of SSI are guaranteed a monthly income of $178 per month or $267 for an eligible couple. Any unearned income (with the exception of the first $20 per month) in excess of the monthly guarantee reduces the SSI benefit dollar for dollar. In addition, monthly wages over $65 reduce the SSI benefit by 50¢ for each dollar of earned income. SSI also imposes a limit on asset holdings of recipients, confining eligibility to individuals whose assets do not exceed $1,500 ($2,250 for couples). Homes, household goods and personal effects, automobiles with a market value under $1,200, and a few other items are excluded from the asset test.

SSI must be viewed as more than a logical and equitable revamping of the existing public assistance programs. In 1973, the year before SSI became effective, there were 1.8 million aged covered by the states' old-age assistance programs. Original estimates projected that the number of aged eligible for the new SSI benefits in January 1974 would increase to 4.9 million or 23 percent of the population age 65 or over. The actual experience was somewhat less dramatic, but there was a significant 36 percent increase in aged beneficiaries to 2.5 million. Most probably this number will grow as more persons become aware of their eligibility under the new program and file for benefits. In addition to the increased number of beneficiaries, the average payment level increased 14 percent with the introduction of SSI. These two factors resulted in an immediate 45 percent growth in welfare expenditures to the aged with the introduction of SSI.

The existence of this federal minimum income guarantee promises to have the most profound impact on the future of Social Security. Since SSI was designed as a floor beneath which no elderly person's income could fall, it can be argued that it weakens the rationale for the welfare or income adequacy role of Social Security, freeing the program to restructure benefits along less progressive lines. The fact that over 70 percent of aged SSI recipients have some income from Social Security suggests that SSI and Social Security are trying to fulfill the same objective for the same target population. However, SSI is a more efficient vehicle for meeting this welfare criterion than Social Security, because a means test ensures that funds actually go to those with a demonstrable need. The progressive Social Security benefits presently distort the contributions-to-benefits schedule in the interests of social adequacy, but actually augment the income of many elderly persons who are relatively well off because of unearned income or a second pension. In effect, many individuals who should be ineligible receive welfare through the Social Security program. This distortion of the social adequacy goal of the Social Security program argues for transferring all welfare provisions for the elderly to the new SSI program.

Employee Retirement Income Security Act of 1974. Just as SSI raises questions about the desirability of increasing Social Security benefits at the low end of the income scale, the growth of the private pension system suggests limiting the extension of benefits at the upper end. In 1974 about 30 million wage and salary workers were covered under private employer-financed retirement plans. Coverage under private plans doubled from 22.5 percent of the labor force to 44.0 percent between 1950 and 1974. Annual contributions to private pensions increased twelvefold from $2 billion in 1950 to $25 billion in 1974. Private pension contributions in 1974 equaled approximately one-half of the $48 billion payroll tax payment to the old-age and survivors insurance trust fund for the same year. By 1974, six million retirees and survivors were actually receiving benefits from private pension plans, compared to 19 million individuals receiving old-age and survivors benefits under Social Security. Beneficiaries of private pension plans were paid a total of $13 billion, which averages out to slightly more than $2,000 per recipient (Table II).

In spite of the rapid growth in private pensions, Congressional investigations in the late 1960s and early 1970s found that many plans were seriously underfunded or mismanaged and that the vesting provisions of some plans were so stringent that they deprived many employees of the retirement income upon which they had based their financial planning. In addition, it was found that many employees lost all rights to a pension when they changed employers or when their firms went bankrupt, were reorganized, or merged.

After years of study, Congress passed the Employee Retirement Income Security Act (ERISA) of 1974, a measure which set up minimum vesting and portability standards for private plans and which created the Pension Benefit Guaranty Corporation, an agency empowered to pay as much as $750 monthly to a retiree whose pension plan fails to meet its obligations. Another provision of the act introduced individual retirement accounts (IRAs) for workers not covered by a company or union plan. Under this scheme, workers may set aside up to 15 percent of their annual income (or $1,500, whichever is less) for retirement, and the

Table II

GROWTH OF PRIVATE PENSIONS, 1950–1974

	Contributions *(millions)*			Benefits		
	Total	*Employer*	*Employee*	*Number of Beneficiaries (thousands)*	*Amount of Payments (millions)*	*Reserves, end of year (billions)*
1950	$ 2,080	$ 1,750	$ 330	450	$ 370	$ 12.1
1955	3,840	3,280	560	980	850	27.5
1960	5,490	4,710	780	1,780	1,720	52.0
1965	8,360	7,370	990	2,750	3,520	86.5
1970	14,000	12,580	1,420	4,740	7,360	137.1
1973	21,100	19,390	1,710	6,080	11,220	180.2
1974	25,020	23,020	2,000	6,390	12,930	191.7

Source: Alfred M. Skolnik, "Private Pension Plans, 1950-74," *Social Security Bulletin*, Vol. 39, No. 6 (June, 1976), p. 4.

contributions to and earnings from the account are tax exempt until the worker retires. At the same time the tax treatment of the self-employed was liberalized; they are now allowed to deduct as much as $7,500 (the previous limit was $2,500) for contributions toward retirement funds.

As a result of the 1974 legislation, middle- and high-income workers can supplement their Social Security benefits through either private pension plans or IRAs. In 1977 a worker who had median taxable earnings ($8,813 in 1976) received a Social Security benefit equivalent to 44.7 percent of preretirement (1975) earnings. According to a 1969–1970 survey of newly entitled OASDHI beneficiaries, a retired male worker receiving a private pension as well as Social Security drew an average additional 25 percent of previous earnings in private pension benefits (Kolodrubetz, 1973). Therefore workers with private pension coverage as well as Social Security are insured against a serious decline in income due to retirement. The availability of these private resources to middle- and high-income workers places a ceiling on the desirable level of compulsory public protection. Large public benefits for this group are unnecessary and can only serve to interfere with private saving initiative.

Social Security and Saving: New Evidence. The negative impact of Social Security on personal saving also offers compelling reasons for restricting benefit increases for middle- and high-income workers and preserving the limit on the taxable wage base used to calculate benefits. The available evidence indicates that workers recognize that they will receive benefits in exchange for their current Social Security taxes and that this guaranteed retirement income enters into their savings plans. To the extent that workers view Social Security as a form of compulsory saving they will tend to save less on their own, thus substituting public for private saving. Two recent empirical studies support the conclusion that Social Security benefits decrease personal saving (Feldstein, 1974; Munnell, 1974).

Under the present pay-as-you-go financing, Social Security contributions are immediately distributed as benefits rather than accumulated in a fund; therefore, a reduction in individual private savings implies a corresponding reduction in total capital accumulation. Future expansion of Social Security benefits for middle- and high-income individuals will surely result in increased substitution of public saving financed on a pay-as-you-go basis for private saving accumulated in funds. This shift will reduce the rate of capital accumulation and the growth of the economy, and therefore it represents another argument for "capping off" the Social Security program.

FINANCIAL DEVELOPMENTS

The second major group of developments that will affect the future of Social Security is comprised of the factors underlying the forecast increase in long-run costs of the present program. The official 1976 projections from the Social Security Administration estimate that the combined employer-employee cost for the old-age, survivors, and disability insurance (OASDI) portion of the program would rise from its present level of 10.6 percent of earnings taxed by Social Security to 28.6 percent of taxable payrolls by the year 2050, if the current benefit structure were retained (Annual Report, 1976). (The present combined OASDI tax rate on employers and employees is 9.9 percent, but this rate fails to cover costs of total benefits.)

The projected cost increases can be attributed to two equally important factors. The first, responsible for about one-half of the projected increase, is the changing demographic structure of the population. Today there are 31 beneficiaries for each 100 workers, whereas in the year 2050 it is estimated that there will be 51 for each 100 workers. With a pay-as-you-go system, an increase in the ratio of beneficiaries to workers implies an inevitable matching increase in costs.

The other half of the forecast deficit is due to an unintended feature of the 1972 Social Security legislation which introduced a double adjustment for inflation into the benefit formula. Additional costs due to this technical flaw have been obviated with the passage of the 1977 Social Security legislation and no longer cloud the real issues in long-run financing. The following sections will first describe the nature of this overindexing problem, then evaluate the new demographic assumptions, and finally indicate the potential impact of the long-run cost increase on the nature of the Social Security program.

Overindexing. The 1972 amendments introduced into the Social Security Act a mechanism whereby the benefit formula was adjusted automatically in response to changes in the cost of living. Unfortunately, this desirable adjustment was marred by a serious technical flaw which overcompensated workers for inflation and made future replacement rates (ratio of benefits to worker's final wage) highly dependent on the exact pattern of future wage and price increases (Thompson, 1974). For example, the wage and price assumptions incorporated in the 1976 official projections of the Social Security Administration (wage growth of 5.75 percent and CPI growth of 4 percent) would result in a rise in benefit protection by nearly 50 percent more than the assumed increase in wages during the next century and, in fact, many future retirees would get benefits higher than any wages they had earned.

Until December 1977 the procedure for making cost-of-living adjustments was to change the factors in the Social Security benefit formula as follows. In January 1976 the formula set an earner's primary benefit equal to roughly 129 percent of the first $110 of average monthly wages (AMW), 47 percent of the next $290, 44 percent of the next $150, and so on through five additional brackets (Table III). Since inflation during 1975 averaged 6.4 percent, the formula was automatically changed in June 1976 so that each individual's benefit was defined as 138 percent (or 1.064 of 129 percent) of the first $110, plus 50 percent (or 1.064 of 47 percent) of the next $290, and so forth for all the brackets in the formula.

This adjustment procedure worked well for those beneficiaries of the Social Security system who are already retired. For these individuals, inflation had no effect on the AMW figure used in their benefit calculations; their average wage remained fixed at the actual level of their past earnings, and monthly benefits increased by the same amount as the cost of living. Thus the pur-

Table III

SOCIAL SECURITY BENEFIT FORMULAS BEFORE AND AFTER COST OF LIVING ADJUSTMENT, 1976

Before Cost of Living Adjustment *January 1976*	*After Cost of Living Adjustment* *June 1976*
129.48% of first $110 of AMW [a]	137.77% of first $110 of AMW [a]
plus 47.10% of next $290	plus 50.11% of next $290
plus 44.01% of next $150	plus 46.83% of next $150
plus 51.73% of next $100	plus 55.04% of next $100
plus 28.77% of next $100	plus 30.61% of next $100
plus 23.98% of next $250	plus 25.51% of next $250
plus 21.60% of next $175	plus 22.98% of next $175
plus 20.00% of next $100	plus 21.28% of next $100

Source: U.S. Social Security Administration, Office of the Actuary.

[a] AMW represents average monthly wage in covered employment.

chasing power of their benefits was maintained at its original level.

At the same time, however, this procedure introduced an unintended overadjustment into the benefit levels of those workers who were due to retire in the future, because those still in the labor force would in the long run get wage increases to compensate for the effects of inflation. As a result of the inflation-induced wage increases, these workers would enjoy higher AMWs as well as an inflation-adjusted benefit formula when it came time for them to retire. In this way the overindexed formula gave future retirees a double benefit increase each time there was an increase in the cost of living. In fact, if inflation rates were constant and there were no offsetting downward effect of rising real wages, future retirees would be compensated twice for inflation, and replacement rates would rise by the rate of price increase.

In actual practice, the impact of the inflation overadjustment was not as dramatic as discussed above because of the effect over time on replacement rates of the progressive benefit formula. As an illustration, consider a long period of zero inflation. In this situation the benefit formula would never change because the conversion factors are adjusted only in response to increases in prices. As real wages rise over time, each successive group of newly retired workers would find themselves in higher brackets of the benefit formula, having smaller percentages of their AMW being replaced by retirement benefits. Eventually most of the AMW would fall into the highest bracket, which implies a lower replacement rate. In the absence of inflation, replacement rates tend to decline over time as wages rise due to the progressivity of the benefit formula.

An overadjustment for inflation will cause replacement rates to rise whenever prices increase; the progressivity of the benefit formula will cause replacement rates to fall whenever real wages rise. The net impact of these two forces on replacement rates depends on whether the wage effect or the price effect is dominant. Table IV presents replacement rates over the next 75 years under alternative assumptions about the rate of increase in wages and prices. These data can be used to demonstrate the impact of the two effects.

Table IV

REPLACEMENT RATES[a] FOR MAN RETIRING AT AGE 65 IN SELECTED CALENDAR YEARS 1975–2050, EARNING MEDIAN TAXABLE EARNINGS IN ALL YEARS

| Calendar Year | Assumed Annual Increases in Real Wages and Prices | | | |
	A Real Wages 1% Prices 4%	B Real Wages 2% Prices 4%	C Real Wages 2% Prices 3%	D Real Wages 2% Prices 2%
1975 [b]	.434	.434	.434	.434
1980	.472	.468	.468	.464
1985	.514	.495	.490	.478
1990	.548	.508	.500	.482
1995	.570	.510	.494	.473
2000	.617	.533	.510	.478
2005	.661	.553	.522	.482
2010	.704	.572	.530	.480
2015	.746	.589	.536	.477
2020	.785	.603	.541	.473
2025	.822	.616	.545	.470
2030	.858	.628	.549	.466
2035	.891	.639	.553	.463
2040	.923	.649	.556	.461
2045	.954	.658	.559	.458
2050	.983	.667	.562	.456

Source: U.S. Social Security Administration. Office of the Actuary.

[a] Replacement rate represents the ratio of the primary insurance amount at award (June of year) to monthly taxable earnings in the year just prior to retirement.

[b] 1975 rates are actual.

The depressing effect of rising wages on replacement rates can be seen by comparing two series with the same rate of price increase but differing rates of wage growth. Series A and B both have the same four percent inflation assumption, but Series A assumes real wage growth of one percent while Series B has real wages rising two percent per year. This one percentage point difference in the rate of wage growth results in significantly lower replacement rates under Series B by the year 2050. In that year the replacement rate with the higher real wage growth is 0.667 compared to 0.983 under the low wage growth assumption—a difference of 47 percent.

Comparing replacement rates under Series B and C illuminates the effect of the overadjustment for inflation. Both series assume that real wages grow at two percent, but the inflation rate is one percentage point higher in B than C .The higher rate of inflation causes the replacement rate to climb to 0.667 by the year 2050 compared to 0.562 under the lower inflation assumption.

The enormous variation in replacement rates under alternative wage and price assumptions was a serious defect because replacement rates should be an expected result of deliberate policy rather than an accidental result of the benefit calculation formula. This is necessary both for intergenerational equity and for accurate actuarial analysis of future costs. Therefore it was essential that the inflation adjustment procedure be modified to yield replacement rates which are predictable over time and avoid excessive increases in long-run costs.

Demographic Changes. The half of the long-term cost increase which results from demographic changes cannot be solved by a technical correction. The ratio of aged to working population is projected to rise dramatically as a result of the declining fertility rate and increasing life expectancy. Since Social Security taxes are used immediately to finance current benefits, any increase in the ratio of beneficiaries to workers requires a compensating increase in the payroll taxes per worker to maintain benefit levels. This section explores the nature of the demographic shifts and their impact on Social Security financing.

Since 1800 there has been a persistent decline in the U.S. fertility rate, although there was a transient deviation from this trend during the 1945–1960 period (see Figure 1). Since 1960 the fertility rate has been cut in half from 3.7 to 1.8 in 1975. The 1976 official projection of the Social Security Administration assumes that the downward trend will be checked at a level of 1.75 in 1977, when a gradual upswing will begin. The projected rate would eventually reach 1.9 in the year 2005, where it would remain constant and generate a slowly declining population.

Figure 1 presents the fertility rates underlying the 1976 Social Security fertility assumptions, the most recent projections of the Census Bureau, and the assumptions incorporated in the report of a recent Senate Panel on Social Security Financing (a group of outside actuaries and economists appointed by the Senate Committee on Finance to provide an independent analysis of the actuarial status of Social Security). The differences in the various fertility rate assumptions have enormous implications for estimates of the size and age structure of the population. In contrast to the Social Security Administration's 1973 fertility assumptions which resulted in estimates of U.S. population growth from 220 million in 1974 to 312 million in the year 2000 and finally 515 million in the year 2050, the comparable figures based on the latest Social Security assumptions are 260 million in the year 2000, a peak of 279 million in 2030 and a decline to 274 million by 2050.

The most significant impact of the alternative fertility assumptions for Social Security, however, is not in the absolute size but in the changing age composition of the population. The ratio of aged population to working-age population has increased from 11.7 aged per 100 persons of working age in 1940, to 18.6 aged per 100 of working age in 1973, and is now projected by the Social Security Administration to rise to about 31.9 aged per 100 of working age by the middle of the next century (Figure 2).

From these projected ratios of aged to working-age population, the Social Security Administration has constructed estimates of the changes in the ratio of workers to beneficiaries.

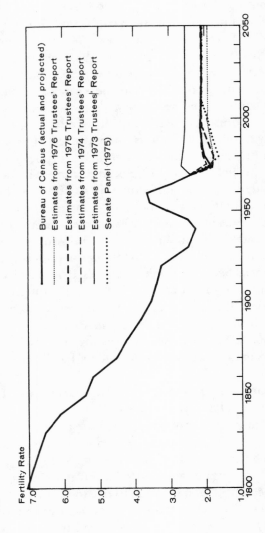

Figure 1 Actual and Projected Fertility Rates in the United States from 1800 to 2050.

Fertility Rate

Bureau of Census (actual and projected)
Estimates from 1976 Trustees' Report
Estimates from 1975 Trustees' Report
Estimates from 1974 Trustees' Report
Estimates from 1973 Trustees' Report
Senate Panel (1975)

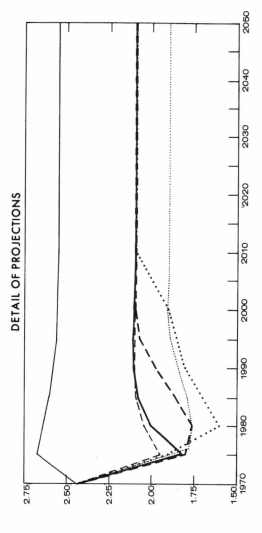

DETAIL OF PROJECTIONS

Sources: Actual rates — 1800-1910, Ansley J. Coale, *New Estimates of Fertility and Population in the U.S.*, Princeton University Press (1963); 1920–1930, National Center for Health Statistics, *Natality Statistics Analysis*, Series 21, No. 19; 1940–1965, Department of Health, Education, and Welfare, *Vital Statistics of the United States* (1969), Vol. 1, Natality (Rockville, Md. 1974), p. 19; 1970, Bureau of the Census, *Current Population Reports, Series P-25, No. 601, p. 126. Project rates — Bureau of the Census, Current Population Reports,* Series P-25, No. 601, p. 126; Social Security Administration, Office of the Actuary, *Population Projections for OASDHI Cost Estimates,* Actuarial Note No. 62 (December 1966), Table 2 (for figures used in 1973 Trustees' Report) and Actuarial Note No. 72, (July 1974), Table 1 (for figures used in 1974 Trustees' Report) and unpublished data (for figures used in 1975 and 1976 Trustees' Report); *Report of the Panel on Social Security Financing to the Committee on Finance of the United States Senate,* 94 Cong., sess. 1 (1975), p. 8.

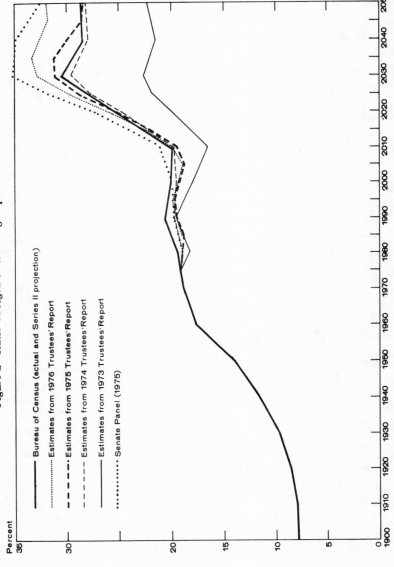

Figure 2 Ratio of Aged to Working Population.

Percent

- — Bureau of Census (actual and Series II projection)
- ········ Estimates from 1976 Trustees' Report
- – – – Estimates from 1975 Trustees' Report
- — — — Estimates from 1974 Trustees' Report
- ——— Estimates from 1973 Trustees' Report
- •••••••• Senate Panel (1975)

There are now 31 beneficiaries for every 100 workers. By the year 2050, with a fertility rate of 1.9 children per woman, there would be 51 beneficiaries for every 100 workers. Under the current method of pay-as-you-go financing, this 65 percent increase in the relative number of beneficiaries requires a 65 percent increase in the OASDI tax rate if benefit replacement rates are to be maintained.

Given the past difficulties in predicting the fertility rate, it is important to try to assess the reliability of the most recent Social Security projections. Demographers generally agree that the present decline in the fertility rate is the continuation of a long-run trend begun in 1800, and that the postwar baby boom was merely a temporary aberration (Mayer, 1974). These expectations are consistent with a series of major developments, all pointing toward smaller families. Information and availability of inexpensive methods of contraception have become more widespread. There has been increased recognition and preference for the higher standard of living made possible in an urbanized society by a smaller family. Furthermore, a variety of factors has contributed to changing the role of women and to their increased desire to participate in the labor force rather than spend long periods at home with children. Finally, zero population growth has become accepted as a desirable social goal.

Although there is general agreement that fertility rates will remain low, there is less consensus about the level around which the rate will eventually stabilize. The 1976 Social Security intermediate cost estimates were based on a fertility rate of 1.9 (alternative cost estimates were also presented based on fertility rates

<hr>

Sources: Actual: Bureau of the Census, 1970 Census of the Population, *Characteristics of the Population, U.S. Summary*, Vol. 1, Part 1, p. 276. Projections: Social Security Administration, Office of the Actuary, *Population Projections for OASDHI Cost Estimates*, Actuarial Note No. 62 (December, 1966) Table 10 (for 1973 Trustees' Report), Actuarial Note No. 76 (July, 1974) Table 10 (for 1974 Trustees' Report); *Annual Report of the Board of Trustees of the Federal Old-Age and Survivors Insurance Trust Funds* (1975), p. 84, (1976), p. 123; Bureau of the Census, *Current Population Reports* Series P–25 (October, 1975) Tables 8 and 11; *Report of the Panel on Social Security Financing to the Committee on Finance of the United States Senate*, 94 Cong., sess 1 (1974), p. 7.

of 1.7 and 2.3) which is considerably below other recent estimates, including the Census Bureau's intermediate projection of a fertility rate of 2.1 beginning around the year 1990 (Figure 1). The higher Census estimate, which corresponds with previous Social Security projections, is buttressed by data from recent surveys of young married women between the ages of 18 and 24 who indicated an average number of expected births of 2.4 in 1971, 2.3 in 1972 and 1973, and 2.2 in 1974. Naturally, after adjustment for those not yet married and those who will remain single, the average fertility rate would be slightly lower. Nevertheless, the fertility rate implied by these recent surveys is closer to the Census figure of 2.1 than the Social Security Administration's latest projection of 1.9. In short, the 1976 Social Security cost estimates may be overly pessimistic because of an unrealistically low estimate of the fertility rate.

Implications of the Projected Deficits. As noted above, the combined impact of the demographic shifts and the overindexing of the benefit formula would have required the Social Security tax rate to be almost triple its present rate by the year 2050. Table V summarizes the increasingly pessimistic long-run projections under the current system and also presents official cost estimates for 1975 and 1976 based on the assumptions that the overindexing was corrected and that replacement rates were stabilized at 1977 and 1978 levels respectively. As discussed earlier, overindexing is an error whose correction precludes capricious replacement rates and undesirable long-run costs, and it should not be allowed to cloud the issues involved in financing the true long-term deficit faced by the system.

Now that the overindexing has been eliminated, the payroll tax rate required to finance benefits in the year 2050 is now projected at 19.2 percent. This 1976 cost estimate for the program without the double inflation adjustment is considerably higher than the comparable 1975 projection, which required a rate of 16.3 percent of taxable payrolls by the year 2050. The higher 1976 cost estimates are derived primarily from the lower fertility rate assumption of 1.9 compared to 2.1 for the 1975 projections and an assumed growth in real wages of 1.75 percent instead of 2 per-

Table V

LONG-RUN PROJECTIONS FOR THE COMBINED OASDI TRUST FUNDS, 1975–2050

Calendar Year	Combined Tax Rate Schedule (Current Law)	Expenditures as a percentage of taxable payroll						
		Present Overindexed System					Revised System	
		1973 Trustees	1974 Trustees	1975 Trustees	1975 Senate Panel	1976 Trustees	1975 Trustees	1976 Trustees
1975[a]	9.9	9.7[b]	10.2	10.9	10.2	10.7	10.9	10.7
1990	9.9	10.0	11.0	11.2	11.5	12.1	11.1	11.9
2010	9.9	10.3	12.7	14.1	14.6	16.0	12.6	13.7
2030	11.9	12.5	17.6	21.8	23.3	26.0	17.2	19.4
2050	11.9	12.6[c]	17.9[c]	22.4	23.9	28.6	16.3	19.2
Average	10.9	10.9	13.9	16.3	16.9	18.9	13.8	15.3
Average Deficit[d]	—	—	3.0	5.3	6.0	8.0	2.9	4.4

Sources: *1973 Annual Report of the Board of Trustees of the Federal Old-Age and Survivors Insurance and Disability Insurance Trust Funds*, Table 18, p. 30; *1974 Annual Report of the Board of Trustees of the Federal Old-Age and Survivors Insurance and Disability Insurance Trust Funds*, Tables 16 and 22, pp. 30 and 37; *1975 Annual Report of the Board of Trustees of the Federal Old-Age and Survivors Insurance and Disability Insurance Trust Funds*, Tables 16, 20, and 24, pp. 49, 60, 71; *Report of the Panel on Social Security Financing, Committee on Finance, U.S. Senate* (Washington, G.P.O., 1975), p. 2; *1976 Annual Report of the Board of Trustees of the Federal Old-Age and Survivors Insurance and Disability Insurance Trust Funds*, Tables 14, 26, and 31, pp. 54, 91 and 107.

[a] Figures from the 1973, 1974, and 1975 Trustees' Reports and from the Senate Panel represent estimates done previous to the actual experience; the figures from the 1976 Trustees' Report are preliminary figures representing the actual experience.

[b] The 1975 figure is actually for 1973.

[c] The 2050 figures is actually for 2045.

[d] The average deficit represents the additional tax required in every year for the system to have sufficient funds to meet total benefit costs and administrative expenses during the next 75 years.

171

cent. Both of these assumptions may be unduly pessimistic, but if they prove correct even the revised system will require a significant increase over the current levy. These projected cost increases for the existing program (even after correcting the overindexing) may create pressure to reduce the scope of Social Security benefits. There are two approaches—one pertaining to the retirement age and one to the level of replacement rates—which if adopted could reduce the long-run financial requirements.

As long as Social Security is financed on a pay-as-you-go basis, future costs will be extremely sensitive to the ratio of retirees to working population, which in turn hinges critically on the retirement age. The projections presented above are based on the assumption that full benefits continue to be awarded at age 65. However the average life expectancy at age 65 increased 25 percent between 1930 and 1970, rising from 12.2 to 15.2 years. Moreover, between 1958 and 1974 the number of days of restricted activity for persons age 65 and over declined 20 percent, dropping from 47.3 to 38.0 days. The large projected deficits and evidence of the increased health and life expectancy of the aged population raise the question of reversing the trend toward early retirement and extending the normal retirement age to 68. Estimates by the Quadrennial Advisory Council on Social Security indicate that if the present retirement age were increased gradually by one month every six months beginning in 2005 and ending in 2023 at age 68, the combined Social Security tax rate could be reduced by 1.5 percentage points by 2050 (Report of the Quadrennial Council, 1975).

Extending the retirement age would simultaneously ease the burden on future taxpayers and bolster the economic welfare of the elderly by shortening the period over which they suffer reduced retirement income. Recent evidence indicates that Social Security has contributed to the trend toward early retirement by introducing actuarially reduced benefits at age 62 and by making receipt of benefits contingent on satisfying an earnings test. Therefore, if it is decided to extend the retirement age, it would be appropriate to eliminate some of the Social Security provisions which discourage labor force participation of the elderly (for example, by either liberalizing the earnings test or increasing the delayed retirement credit).

The second assumption embedded in the long-run cost projections shown in Table V is that the overindexing will be corrected in a fashion that not only stabilizes replacement rates but in fact ensures constant replacement rates over time. These dual objectives were achieved by the recent social security legislation. Replacement rates for workers retiring after 1983 will stabilize at 43 percent, slightly below the current rate. A reasonable alternative would have been to devise a benefit formula which, while making replacement rates independent of the future path of price and wage increases, would allow the ratio of benefits to preretirement earnings to decline gradually over time. An extreme version of this approach would be simply to maintain the real purchasing power of today's benefits. Constant real benefits combined with rising real wages would result in rapidly declining replacement rates and tax rates below current levels. A rationale for this type of strategy would be that present benefit levels allow retired workers to meet their minimum needs and that the goal of Social Security should be merely to continue satisfying these basic needs through adjusting benefit levels over time for rising prices. In the future, individuals could supplement their retirement incomes through private saving out of higher real wages. Declining replacement rates would allow Social Security to provide a floor of income support while reducing the long-run financial requirements of the program. In fact, the Consultant Panel on Social Security has recently proposed a price indexing scheme which would result in a gradual decline in replacement rates that enables tax rates to remain roughly at current levels (Report of the Consultant Panel, 1976).

The long-term financial requirements of the Social Security program are relatively manageable now that the double inflation adjustment has been eliminated. Furthermore, cost estimates for a revised system have been based on the assumption of constant replacement rates over time and full benefits awarded at age 65. If the inevitable increase in cost due to shifting demography is considered excessive, measures can be taken to reduce the financial requirements either by allowing replacement rates to decline or by extending the retirement age or both.

THE BENEFIT STRUCTURE

The benefit structure has required immediate attention because of the overindexing introduced in the 1972 legislation. In the process of developing a new scheme, attention should have been given to the implications of the new Supplemental Security Income (SSI) program for the progressivity of the benefit formula and the minimum benefit, and to the implications of the increased labor force participation of women for dependents' benefits.

SSI and the Progressivity of the Benefit Formula. As shown in Table 3, the benefit formula for 1976 consists of eight brackets in which the percentage of earnings replaced decreases as average earnings increase. The formula is structured so that low-wage workers receive benefits that are a higher proportion of their preretirement earnings than do high-wage workers. Viewed in a lifetime framework, the progressivity implies a disproportionately high rate of return on the contributions of low-income workers. As part of the new indexing scheme, a benefit formula that closely duplicates the existing structure was designed. However, the issue of the appropriate "tilt" or progressivity of the formula should be given serious consideration as it may not be the appropriate policy for the future.

Some advocates of a progressive benefit formula base their arguments on the fact that the existing overall distribution is unsatisfactory and that Social Security expenditures should be used to achieve a more equitable result. Since benefit payments for OASDI currently account for almost 20 percent of the federal budget, they feel there is no reason to exempt such a large expenditure from the redistributive effort.

On the other hand, redistribution through the Social Security benefit structure is inefficient. Individuals receive disproportionately high benefits regardless of whether their low average earnings are attributable to low wage rates or simply to short periods in covered employment. Thus many of the progressive benefits simply go to the beneficiaries of other government pension programs who have spent a minimum period in covered industry. In addition, Social Security imposes no means or asset tests, paying equal amounts to those with substantial savings and those with no other source of income. Redistribution could be accomplished more efficiently by channeling funds to low-income families through an expanded means-tested Supplemental Security Income (SSI) program and by returning Social Security to a wage-related benefit system. With this approach, funds would be directed to individuals who are poor rather than to those who simply have experienced low earnings in covered employment but have other sources of income.

Another argument favoring a progressive benefit formula can be couched in the context of the goals of the Social Security program itself, rather than in terms of the overall distribution of income. To prevent a serious decline in income upon retirement, retirees require about 70 percent of their gross preretirement earnings. (This low percentage reflects the decline in work-related expenses, the tax-free status of some retirement income, and the health insurance available to the elderly. See Table VI.) Guaranteeing all workers 70 percent of their previous earnings in retirement would be very expensive and would require almost double the present payroll taxes. The pragmatic compromise, therefore, is to provide higher replacement rates for low-income workers who cannot save on their own, and lower replacement rates for high-income workers who can supplement their benefits with private pensions and saving.

However there are two possible methods of achieving a system of progressive replacement rates. On the one hand, the present Social Security benefit structure could be retained, with its minimum benefit provision and steeply progressive benefit formula. The alternative would be to provide proportional benefits to all retirees through the Social Security program, combined with supplementary benefits for low-income workers provided by SSI. This approach would completely separate the goals of earnings

Table VI

CALCULATION OF RETIREMENT INCOME EQUIVALENT TO PRERETIREMENT INCOME FOR MARRIED COUPLES RETIRING JANUARY, 1976—VARIOUS INCOME LEVELS

Item	Levels of Income					
Preretirement Income	$4,000	$6,000	$8,000	$10,000	$15,000
Federal Income Tax[a]	28	330	679	1,059	2,002
Federal OASDHI Tax[b]	234	351	468	585	824
Preretirement Income After Federal Personal Taxes	3,738	5,319	6,853	8,356	12,174
State Income Tax[c] (13.1 percent of Federal)	4	43	89	139	262
Preretirement Disposable Income After Federal and State Personal Taxes	3,734	5,276	6,763	8,217	11,912
Savings Resulting from Retirement[d]	544	816	1,088	1,360	2,040
Retirement Income Needed to Equal Preretirement Disposable Income:[e] Amount	3,190	4,460	5,675	6,857	9,872
Percent of Preretirement Total Income	80	74	71	69	66

Sources: Commerce Clearing House, Inc. *1976 Federal Tax Return Manual* (Washington, 1976), pp. 103, 107, 108. U.S. Department of Labor "Revised Equivalence Scale for Estimating Equivalent Incomes or Budget Costs by Family Type," *Bureau of Labor Statistics Bulletin* No. 1570–2, 1968, Table 1. State income tax as percent of Federal income tax figures from income tax receipt estimates given by U.S. Department of Commerce, Bureau of Economic Analysis.

[a]Calculated in accord with prevailing tax code.

[b]For 1975, 5.85 percent on earnings up to $14,100.

[c]In 1974 state (and local) income tax receipts were 13.1 percent of Federal income tax receipts. This percentage probably rose in 1975 because Federal taxes were decreased while state taxes increased. Therefore, the percent of preretirement income needed to maintain living standards is probably slightly overstated.

[d]Savings from retirement are based on the "Revised Equivalence Scale for Estimating Equivalent Income or Budget Costs by Family Type" (*BLS Bulletin* No. 1570–2, 1968). Consumption requirements for a two person husband-wife family after retirement are 86.4 percent of those for a like family prior to retirement (age 55–64). Savings are therefore estimated at 13.6 percent of preretirement income.

[e]It can be assumed that retirement income for these income classes will not be subject to taxes.

replacement and income maintenance into two programs. The earnings replacement function would be performed by Social Security as a strictly wage-related system with replacement rates equal across all earnings levels. The income support function would be transferred to SSI, which is financed by the progressive income tax. The advantages of this approach are significant.

Shifting the welfare function to SSI would rationally redistribute, though not necessarily reduce, the total financial burden of income maintenance for the aged. A proportional Social Security program would establish a logical basis on which to separate the financing of earnings replacement and welfare. Social Security benefits would be strictly related to past contributions and therefore appropriately financed by the payroll tax. All supplementary payments to low-income individuals under SSI would be financed by high-income individuals through the personal income tax. This transfer would be more effective than the present scheme whereby the progressive benefits provided to the elderly through Social Security are financed by low- and middle-income workers through the regressive payroll tax.

Second, a proportional Social Security benefit structure would ensure that all future workers receive a positive return on their contribution. In the past, the expansion of coverage and the growing labor force have provided adequate revenues to provide a positive return to all workers and while pursuing the goal of social adequacy through a progressive benefit structure. However, coverage is now virtually complete (with the exception of federal employees and some state and local workers) and population growth is expected to cease; therefore, the real rate of return on Social Security contributions will tend toward the rate of growth of real wages, or about two percent. In fact, the working age population is actually scheduled to decline, and this decline will reduce the return below its equilibrium rate of two percent. In this setting, the goals of a fair return and social adequacy come into direct conflict, because a steeply progressive benefit structure will probably yield negative returns to workers with above-average earnings. Once this happened, support for the Social Security program might decline.

Furthermore, to the extent that workers perceive the Social Security levy as another tax reducing take-home wages, this tax will have a discouraging effect on labor force participation, particularly of secondary workers. If the tax were clearly identified as merely a compulsory saving, workers may perceive their contribution as part of their net wage. This change in perceptions would eliminate any existing distortions on work effort.

Finally, if benefits were strictly proportional to contributions, it would be possible for legislation to give individuals the alternative of "opting out" of the Social Security program (perhaps with some penalty), provided they accumulated funds for retirement elsewhere. Those indviduals who chose to save outside of the Social Security system would contribute to private capital formation.

Table VII presents a simple example of how a proportional benefit structure could be combined with an expanded SSI program to guarantee adequate protection to all retirees and supplemental benefits to low-income individuals. In the example, Social Security benefits are set at 40 percent of preretirement earnings, approximately equivalent to the current replacement rate for workers with median earnings. The example is also based on an expanded Supplemental Security Income program wherein the SSI payment is reduced by only 50¢ for each dollar of Social Security benefits, rather than the present dollar for dollar reduction. With this reduced rate the $20 disregard for Social Security benefits has been eliminated. This reduction in the implicit tax on Social Security would naturally raise the cost of SSI, but a proportional Social Security system is not desirable unless low-income individuals can be adequately protected by such a means-tested program. Reducing the implicit tax would extend assistance to persons through the median income level, thereby insulating all low-wage earners who now gain income from the progressive Social Security benefit structure from a decline in retirement income by the introduction of a proportional benefit formula. Furthermore, reducing the SSI tax rate on Social Security benefits would also ensure that individuals receive some payoff for a lifetime of payroll taxes and would eliminate some serious horizontal inequities between individuals who qualify for SSI and those who must rely on Social Security, by making the cutoff point for SSI less abrupt.

SSI, Dual Beneficiaries, and the Minimum Benefit.   A $10 minimum benefit was introduced in 1939 primarily for reasons of administrative efficiency. Over time, in response to criticism that the minimum benefit was inadequate to meet basic needs, the minimum has grown more than twice as fast as average benefits. Recently, however, there have been suggestions that the minimum benefit be gradually elminated. Among those calling for its elimination was the 1975 Social Security Advisory Council. Although the minimum benefit may have performed a useful role in reducing poverty among the aged in the past, it can be argued that the enactment of the SSI program has eliminated the need for Social Security to include social welfare objectives within its earnings-related benefit program. Furthermore, there is increasing evidence that a large portion of very low benefits are being paid to individuals who were not primarily dependent on earnings in covered employment during their working years and are not primarily dependent on Social Security benefits during their retirement years.

Minimum benefits are currently payable on the basis of average monthly earnings under Social Security of $76 or less. Earnings of this level suggest very weak attachment to the labor force, since a man retiring at age 65 in January 1976 who worked throughout his life at the prevailing minimum wage would have average monthly earnings of $262.40. Under the present system, workers entitled to other major pensions such as federal civil service retirement benefits can easily achieve insured status (10 years or 40 quarters) under Social Security and receive the minimum benefit in addition to their regular pension. The extent to which dual benefits are received is considerable. It was estimated in 1968 that approximately 40 percent of those receiving civil service retirement benefits were also receiving Social Security benefits (Storey, 1973). The minimum benefit thus often serves to supplement the income of those relatively more affluent retirees who receive other pensions, in direct conflict with its stated

Table VII

COMPARISON OF BENEFIT LEVELS AND REPLACEMENT RATES FOR MALES RETIRING AT
AGE 65 IN JANUARY 1976 UNDER PRESENT AND PROPOSED SYSTEMS

Earnings [a]	Monthly [b] Earnings 1975	Present System				
		Social Security Benefit	Replacement Rate	SSI Benefit	Combined Benefit	Combined Replacement Rate
60% of Minimum Wage	$219.00	$165.50	.756	$12.20	$177.70	.811
Low [c]	286.58	178.50	.623	0	178.50	.623
Lower Middle [d]	487.25	238.20	.489	0	238.20	.489
Median	687.92	298.50	.434	0	298.50	.434
Higher Middle [e]	931.46	329.30	.353	0	329.30	.353
High	1,175.00	364.00	.310	0	364.00	.310

Proposed Proportional Benefit System

Earnings [a]	Monthly [b] Earnings 1975	Social Security Benefit	Replacement Rate	SSI Benefit 50% Implicit Tax, no $20 Deductible	Combined Benefit	Combined Replacement Rate
60% of Minimum Wage	$219.00	$ 87.60	.400	$113.90	$201.50	.920
Low [c]	286.58	114.63	.400	100.39	215.02	.750
Lower Middle [d]	487.25	194.90	.400	60.25	255.15	.523
Median	687.92	275.17	.400	20.11	295.28	.429
Higher Middle [e]	931.46	372.58	.400	0	372.58	.400
High	1,175.00	470.00	.400	0	470.00	.400

Source: Committee on Finance of the United States Senate, *The Social Security Act (As Amended Through July 1975), and Related Laws* (Washington: 1975) pp. 124-127.

[a] It is assumed that these individuals enjoyed a smooth income growth each year.
[b] Upon retirement at age 65 in 1976 these persons' career AMWs as calculated by the Social Security Administration would be $157, $184, $313, $442, $514 and $586 respectively.
[c] Represents a person steadily employed at slightly below the minimum wage to reflect the earnings of the large number of workers covered by Social Security who are not affected by Federal standards.
[d] Represents a person whose income is exactly midway between Low and Median.
[e] Represents a person whose income is exactly midway between Median and High.

welfare objective. The minimum benefit should be phased out because it has not been an efficient welfare device, is not consistent with a wage-related benefit structure, and with the advent of SSI is no longer needed to achieve social adequacy.

Working Women and Dependents' Benefits. In most married couples today, both the husband and the wife work. In March 1975, there were 37.4 million families in which the husband was between ages 25 and 65. Of these families, 18.0 million, or 48 percent, were families in which both the husband and wife were in the labor force (U.S. Bureau of the Census, 1977). The trend of increased labor force participation by women implies that in the future a large majority will be covered under Social Security on the basis of their own earnings records. By 1970, 68 percent of women 45–49 years of age already had enough quarters of covered work to be insured for their own primary benefit (Reno, 1973). Estimates for the year 2020 predict that about 70 percent of all aged wives of retired worker beneficiaries will be entitled to benefits on the basis of their own earnings records (Report of the Advisory Council, 1975).

Furthermore, dependents' benefits are the source of many inequities of the Social Security program. The difficulties arise because the beneficiary unit and the taxpaying unit are not the same. That is, the tax is levied on the individual, while the beneficiary unit is the family. Compare two workers retiring at age 65 with identical earnings histories, one single and one married with a spouse aged 65. Both workers pay the same amount in taxes and receive equal primary benefits; however, the married worker receives an additional 50 percent of the primary benefit for support of his spouse. This extra retirement income substantially raises the wage replacement rate for the married worker. In other words, a married worker receives more Social Security benefits for his payroll tax dollar than does a single worker.

The most serious inequity arises in the case of two-earner families, when the wife contributes to the Social Security system through the payroll tax on her earnings but receives the wife's benefit based on her husband's earnings record (if it is greater than the benefit she would receive from her own earnings record). Thus the two-worker family can contribute the same amount as an identical family with a nonworking wife but receive less in benefits. For example, consider two families with identical total earnings. In family A, the husband and wife have each earned 50 percent of the maximum taxable amount in effect in each year. If both retired at age 65 in January 1976, the husband would receive a monthly benefit of $229.20 while the wife would receive $235.80. (The discrepancy in amounts is the result of the shorter computation period for women. This discrepancy is being corrected.) Thus total family benefits would be $465.00. In family B, the husband has earned the maximum taxable amount in all years while the wife has not worked. If he retired at age 65 in January 1976, family B would receive benefits totaling $546.00 (150 percent of the husband's primary benefit). Thus, although both families contributed the same amount, the one-earner family would receive $972.00 more per year in benefits than the two-earner family.

The increased self-reliance of women and the inequities in the system which result from differential treatment of single versus married and one-earner versus two-earner families raise the question of phasing out the secondary retirement benefits of aged spouses. However, if it is decided that dependents' benefits should be eliminated, some provision must be made for the retirement income of aged women who do not participate in the labor force. Mandatory division of a married couple's contribution credits is one possible solution. Such an arrangement would provide a permanent earnings base for the wife, thereby entitling her to benefits in her own right. Another alternative is to have the married workers contribute 150 percent of the tax paid by a single worker in order to guarantee a supplementary 50 percent benefit for a nonworking spouse.

Phasing out secondary benefits would eliminate adult dependency as a criterion for receiving benefits, would move Social Security toward a wage-related system, and would reduce long-run costs. The largest savings would begin to be realized just after the turn of the century, at the same time that the actuarial deficit is projected to increase sharply because of demographic shifts.

THE PAYROLL TAX

All the recent developments—the introduction of SSI, the increase in dual beneficiaries, and the trend in labor force participation by women—suggest a movement toward a more strictly wage-related benefit program. Such a shift in the relative importance of individual equity compared to social adequacy would have significant implications for the continuing acceptability of the payroll tax as a source of financing. The new earned income credit also makes the payroll tax more attractive because this provision eliminates the tax burden on some low-income families.

The issue of the payroll tax for financing Social Security is particularly important because this tax is not only the second largest source of revenue but also the fastest growing. The Social Security payroll tax was introduced in 1935 to finance a system of retirement benefits. The initial rate was 1 percent payable by employees and employers on the first $3,000 of wage income beginning in 1937. By 1977 the payroll tax rate for retirement, survivor's, and disability benefits had risen to 4.95 percent for both employers and employees on the first $16,500 of wage income, with the ceiling scheduled to rise automatically with the wage level. Hospital insurance contributions raised the overall OASDHI payroll tax rate to 5.85 percent. Table VIII summarizes the changes in tax base and rates since the beginning of the program.

As shown in Table 9, total OASDHI receipts in 1975 amounted to almost $76 billion, representing more than a sixfold increase since 1960. The growth in dollar receipts of the Social Security payroll tax has been paralleled by its growing importance as a revenue source. In 1950 the Social Security tax accounted for only 5 percent of all Federal receipts, but its share has doubled every 10 years since then, so that in 1975 the OASDHI taxes raised more than 25 percent of Federal revenues—second in importance only to the personal income tax.

The Earned Income Credit. Like all payroll taxes, the Social Security tax is very regressive, forcing low-income individuals to contribute a disproportionately large share of the revenue. The regressivity can be attributed to two underlying facets of this tax. First, the tax is levied only on wage income, thus excluding all income from capital, a source whose importance increases as income increases. Second, all wages above the maximum taxable limit—$16,500 in 1977—are excluded from Social Security taxation.

For low-income familes with children, the OASDHI payroll tax is now partially offset by the earned income credit, a feature introduced into the personal income tax by the Tax Reduction Act of 1975. This credit, which is available only to low-income workers who have dependent children and maintain a household, amounts to 10 percent of the first $4,000 of earned income, after which the credit is reduced by 10 percent of the taxpayer's adjusted gross income in excess of $4,000. The effect of the credit is to reduce the OASDI portion of the Social Security tax (9.9 percent of taxable payroll under the assumption that labor also bears the employer's portion of the tax either through lower wages or through higher prices) to zero for eligible families with incomes less than $4,000. The OASDI tax then becomes progressive as a percentage of wages between $4,000 and $8,000, proportional between $8,000 and $15,300, and regressive thereafter.

Individual Equity and the Payroll Tax. Although the earned income credit relieves the excessive burden on the poor, the overall acceptability of the OASDI payroll tax depends on the deeper issue of the intended effect of the Social Security program on the distribution of income. With the steeply progressive benefit formula, minimum benefit, and benefits for dependents, some have argued that Social Security is best construed as an annual tax-transfer program which redistributes income from the relatively affluent workers to the poorer retired population (Pechman, Aaron & Taussig, 1968). The alternative perspective

Table VIII

HISTORY OF CONTRIBUTION RATES, MAXIMUM AMOUNT OF TAXABLE EARNINGS, AND MAXIMUM TAX PER YEAR, 1937 to 1976, AND PRESENTLY SCHEDULED CHANGES TO 2011

Calendar years	Maximum Taxable Earnings	Contribution Rates (Percentage of Taxable Earnings) Employees and employers, each				Maximum Possible Tax per year Employees and Employers, each
		OASDHI	OASI	DI	HI	
Past experience:						
1937-49	$3,000	1.000	1.000	—	—	$30.00
1950	3,000	1.500	1.500	—	—	45.00
1951-53	3,600	1.500	1.500	—	—	54.00
1954	3,600	2.000	2.000	—	—	72.00
1955-56	4,200	2.000	2.000	—	—	84.00
1957-58	4,200	2.250	2.000	0.250	—	94.50
1959	4,800	2.500	2.250	.250	—	120.00
1960-61	4,800	3.000	2.750	.250	—	144.00
1962	4,800	3.125	2.875	.250	—	150.00
1963-65	4,800	3.625	3.375	.250	—	174.00
1966	6,600	4.200	3.500	.350	0.350	277.20
1967	6,600	4.400	3.550	.350	.500	290.40
1968	7,800	4.400	3.325	.475	.600	343.20
1969	7,800	4.800	3.725	.475	.600	374.40
1970	7,800	4.800	3.650	.550	.600	374.40

1971	7,800	5.200	4.050	.550	.600	405.60
1972	9,000	5.200	4.050	.550	.600	468.00
1973	10,800	5.850	4.300	.550	1.000	631.80
1974	13,200	5.850	4.375	.575	.900	772.20
1975	14,100	5.850	4.375	.575	.900	824.85
1976	15,300	5.850	4.375	.575	.900	895.05

Changes scheduled in present law:

1977[a]	16,500[b]	5.850	4.375	.575	.900	965.25[c]
1978	17,700[b]	6.050	4.350	.600	1.100	1070.85[c]
1979	19,200[b]	6.050	4.350	.600	1.100	1161.60[c]
1980	21,000[b]	6.050	4.350	.600	1.100	1270.50[c]
1981	22,800[b]	6.300	4.300	.650	1.350	1436.40[c]
1982-1985	—	6.300	4.300	.650	1.350	—
1986-2010	—	6.450	4.250	.700	1.500	—
2011+	—	7.450	5.100	.850	1.500	—

Sources: *1976 Annual Report of the Board of Trustees of the Federal Old-Age and Survivors Insurance and Disability Insurance Trust Funds*, pp. 13, 43; *1974 Annual Report of the Board of Trustees of the Federal Hospital Insurance Trust Fund*, p.5.

[a] 1977 on — subject to automatic revisions.
[b] Estimate from the *1976 Annual Report of the Board of Trustees of the Federal Old-Age and Survivors Insurance and Disability Insurance Trust Funds*, p. 43.
[c] 1977 on — dependent on maximum taxable amount of annual earnings.

Table IX
FEDERAL TAX RECEIPTS, CALENDAR YEARS 1935-1975
(billions of dollars)

	1935	1940	1950	1960	1970	1975
Total Receipts	4.0	8.6	49.9	96.5	192.1	283.5
Personal Income Tax	0.8	1.4	18.1	43.6	92.2	125.6
Payroll Tax	0.1	2.0	5.9	17.7	49.7	93.5
Social Security						
OASDHI	—	0.3	2.7	11.9	39.7	75.6
OASI	—	0.3	2.7	10.9	30.3	56.8
DI	—	—	—	1.0	4.5	7.3
HI	—	—	—	—	4.9	11.5
Other [a]	0.1	1.7	3.2	5.8	10.0	17.9
Corporate Income Tax	0.8	2.6	17.0	21.7	30.8	40.2
Indirect Business and						
Non-Tax Receipts	2.2	2.6	8.9	13.5	19.3	24.2

Sources: *Social Security Bulletin, Annual Statistical Supplement, 1973,* Tables 31-33 pp. 61-63; *Social Security Bulletin,* Vol. 39, (June 1976), Table M-4; *Economic Report of the President,* January 1976, Table B-67, p. 250; U.S. Department of Commerce, *The National Income and Product Accounts of the United States, 1929-1965, Statistical Tables,* (Washington, D.C., G.P.O., 1966), p. 52.

[a] Such as receipts allocated to the unemployment insurance trust fund, the railroad retirement fund, the Federal civil service retirement fund or the veterans' life insurance fund.

is to view Social Security in a lifetime framework in which payroll taxes are considered compulsory saving for retirement.

The annual view of Social Security, as one component of the federal government's tax and transfer schemes, leads to an evaluation of the Social Security payroll tax independent of benefits. The inevitable conclusion is that the Social Security payroll tax clearly violates the ability-to-pay criterion for equitable taxation. The tax is levied without provision for number of dependents, it taxes only wages, and it exempts wages over the maximum. The earned income credit goes part of the way toward eliminating the burden on the working poor. However, this credit is limited to taxpayers with children and therefore provides no relief for low-income childless couples or for single individuals.

An annual tax-transfer perspective naturally leads to favoring a more progressive source of revenue. Benefits for the aged should be financed by the most equitable and progressive levy—namely, the personal income tax. Indeed once the annual perspective is adopted, the Social Security payroll tax, even modified by an expanded earned income credit and with no limit on taxable earnings, must be judged inferior to the personal income tax.

An annual perspective, however, seems at variance with even the existing structure of the Social Security program. The Social Security system is inappropriate as an annual redistributive scheme because it transfers funds to all covered retirees irrespective of need and has traditionally collected a large portion of its revenues from low-income workers. It is extremely difficult to argue for this type of insurance structure on the grounds of annual redistributive goals. If the system were simply part of society's overall redistributive program, then it should be restructured in line with an expanded SSI financed by general revenues.

In fact, the present system can best be understood when considered in the framework of a lifetime compulsory saving. Social Security is a device to force individuals to save during their working years to ensure adequate income in retirement. The payroll tax with an earned income credit is an appropriate method of financing a compulsory savings program. This would be espe-cially true if the program functioned on the basis of an individual equity criterion and phased out the minimum benefit, depen-dents' benefits, and the steeply progressive benefit formula. However, the earned income credit is an essential ingredient to the acceptability of the payroll tax, because compulsory saving schemes simply do not make sense for low-income families. It is unreasonable to impose payroll taxes on poor families whose incomes are considered too meager to support personal income taxes and then to justify those taxes on the grounds that they will receive retirement benefits two or three decades hence. These poor families cannot afford to save, and therefore forcing them to contribute to a Social Security program will compel them to borrow at extremely high market interest rates. Accumulating their Social Security contributions at a real rate of interest of two or three percent while they must borrow at rates in excess of 10 percent cannot be viewed as distributionally neutral. Fortunately, the earned income credit—once it is expanded to include all low-income families—provides a nice solution to the burden of the Social Security payroll tax on low-wage workers.

CONCLUSION

The Social Security system faces a challenge involving changes in the basic nature of the system. The more immediate problem of correction of the "overindexing" of benefits in order to stabi-lize replacement rates has been resolved. The longer-run ques-tion is whether Social Security could better meet the needs of the American people by becoming a pure wage-related annuity pro-gram.

Traditionally, Social Security has combined the goals of indi-vidual equity and social adequacy. Benefits have been related to earnings, but the relationship has been modified to provide an adequate level of income support to the low-income retired pop-ulation. Social adequacy has been reflected in the progressive benefit structure, the minimum benefit, and benefits for dependents and survivors. In the past the trade-off between individual equity and social adequacy was necessary and desirable. However recent developments all raise the question of whether Social Security should become a strictly wage-related benefit program.

The Supplemental Security Income program, enacted in 1972, relieves the need for Social Security to function as a welfare system by providing a federally guaranteed floor beneath which an aged person's income may not fall. Similarly, the Employee Retirement Income Security Act of 1974 ensures the availability of private resources to middle- and high-income workers by regulating and promoting the development of private pensions. New evidence that provision of public retirement benefits depresses the rate of capital accumulation by interfering with private saving initiatives reinforces the need for a ceiling on the level of compulsory public protection. Limited by SSI and private saving mechanisms, Social Security can now fulfill a more precisely defined role in a broader retirement income program by ensuring the primary portion of earnings-related retirement benefits to the majority of the working population.

Within this second tier of earnings-related benefits, recent developments suggest restoring individual equity as the primary criterion. The introduction of SSI, together with the increased labor force participation by women, paves the way for eliminating benefits for dependents and the minimum benefit. Elimination of dependents' benefits will (1) restore equity between single versus married, and one-earner versus two-earner families; (2) make benefits more directly related to individual contributions; and (3) reduce long-run costs. Abolishing the minimum benefit will also lower costs and eliminate the windfall to beneficiaries of other government pension programs who attain minimum coverage under Social Security.

The next step to restore complete individual equity to the Social Security program would be to substitute a proportional benefit formula for the present progressive structure. Low-income individuals would still be treated favorably since they receive an earned income credit, introduced in the Tax Reduction Act of 1975, which offsets their OASDI contributions. Retirees with very low benefits could also apply for income supplementation under the SSI program.

The relative importance of individual equity compared to social adequacy has significant implications for the method by which the system should be financed. As long as the goals of income redistribution and earnings replacement are combined, the payroll tax must be viewed separately from future benefits and evaluated on its own merits. The payroll tax taken by itself is clearly regressive and an inappropriate means of financing a redistributive system. However, if individual equity were restored to the system and benefits were directly related to a worker's contributions, then Social Security taxes could be viewed as a form of compulsory saving which was returned to the worker in his old age. In a strictly wage-related benefit system, the payroll tax is quite an acceptable basis for collecting contributions.

One important question remains: should benefits be contingent upon withdrawal from the labor force, or should they be awarded as annuities at a certain age? Although the retirement test has been criticized extensively, officials of the Social Security Administration have argued that it would be inconsistent with the earnings-replacement function of the program to award benefits while individuals continued to work. This goal of Social Security must be re-evaluated in light of recent evidence that Social Security discourages the elderly from working. If Social Security were a wage-related benefit program which promoted individual equity, benefits should be awarded at a given age regardless of labor force status. Eliminating the retirement test would thus allow older individuals to remain in the work force and would encourage later retirement. Reversing the current trend toward earlier retirement would also open up the possibility of gradually extending the age at which full benefits are awarded from 65 to perhaps 68. Later entitlement would significantly reduce long-run costs, which are scheduled to triple by the middle of the next century.

The Social Security program is at the most critical juncture of its 40-year life. If Social Security is going to be responsive to the changing social structure, the program must be revamped to reflect the introduction of SSI and the existence of the private pension system, to adapt to the evolving nature of the family and the increased labor force participation by women, and to recognize the new economic evidence on saving and retirement. Social Security is an enormous program and its future must be carefully planned, for it will have a significant impact on all aspects of the economy.

REFERENCES

Annual Report of the Board of Trustees of the Federal Old-Age and Survivors Insurance and Disability Insurance Trust Funds. Unpublished report. Washington, D.C.: Social Security Administration, 1976.

Feldstein, M. Social Security, induced retirement, and aggregate capital accumulation. *Journal of Political Economy,* 1974, *82,* 906–926.

Kolodrubetz, W. W. Private retirement benefits and relationship to earnings: Survey of new beneficiaries. *Social Security Bulletin,* 1973, *36* (5), 16–36.

Mayer, L. A. It's a bear market for babies, too. *Fortune,* 1974, *90,* 134–137.

Munnell, A. H. *The effect of Social Security on personal saving.* Cambridge, Mass.: Ballinger, 1974.

Pechman, J. A., Aaron, H. J. & Taussig, M. K. *Social Security: Perspectives for reform.* Washington, D.C.: The Brookings Institution, 1968.

Reno, V. Women newly entitled to retired-worker benefits: Survey of new beneficiaries. *Social Security Bulletin,* 1973, *36*(4), 3–26.

Reports of the Advisory Council on Social Security. Unpublished report. Washington, D.C.: Social Security Administration, 1975.

Report of the Consultant Panel on Social Security to the United States Congressional Research Service, April 1976. Washington, D.C.: U.S. Government Printing Office, 1976.

Report of the Quadrennial Advisory Council on Social Security. Washington, D.C.: Social Security Administration, 1975.

Storey, J. R. Public income transfer programs: The incidence of multiple benefits and the issues raised by their receipt. Prepared for the Subcommittee on Fiscal Policy of the Joint Economic Committee. *Studies in Public Welfare,* Paper No. 1. 93 Cong., 1 Sess., 1973.

Thompson, L. H. An analysis of the factors currently determining benefit level adjustments in the Social Security retirement program. *Technical Analysis Paper No. 1.* Washington, D. C.: Office of Income Security Policy, U.S. Department of HEW, 1974.

Thompson, L. H. An analysis of the issues involved in securing constant replacement rates in the Social Security OASDI program. *Technical Analysis Paper No. 5*. Washington, D. C.: Office of Income Security Policy, U.S. Department of HEW, 1975.

U.S. Bureau of the Census. Consumer Income. *Current Population Reports, Series P-60, No. 97*. Washington, D.C.: U.S. Government Printing Office, January 1975.

-6-

The Future of Private and Public Employee Pensions

Francis P. King

Slightly less than half (46 percent) of all workers in the private sector are now employed by firms having a pension plan. However, provisions for delay in the vesting of plan benefits effectively exclude many workers from ultimately receiving pension benefits, because workers who change jobs or leave for other reasons gain no credit from prevested periods of plan membership. At the same time, over 90 percent of employees in the public sector (workers for federal, state, or local government) are covered by pension plans. Here also, delays in vesting affect ultimate benefits, but lower turnover in the public sector reduces the numbers of employees affected.

Although private retirement plans have grown rapidly in the last 35 years, they clearly have not reached their maximum potential as a part of the total income-support system for the aged. In considering policy questions related to adequate income support in old age, it is important to evaluate the future role that can be played by the private pension system. The purpose of this chapter is to discern the trends that in the past have brought private pensions to their present stage as providers of income for the elderly, to assess the possible effects of expected demographic, economic, and social change on private pensions, and to identify policies that may in the future have a positive effect on the capabilities of private pension plans.

This chapter first offers some basic definitions required for a discussion of employee pension plans, and briefly traces the growth and development of these plans. It then discusses the influence of public policy through legislation, in particular the Pension Reform Act of 1974. A resumé of the characteristics of present employee pension plans is followed by a discussion of the possible effects of future demographic, economic, and social changes.

Definitions. The funding of private pensions must be distinguished from the funding methods of the Social Security program, which is a social transfer system. Under Social Security, current workers are taxed to provide funds for immediate transfer to current beneficiaries, including retired persons and their dependents, survivors of workers and their dependents, and disabled workers and their dependents. In contrast, private pensions are built on the principle of reserve funding. Invested funds and fund earnings are accumulated and form the present value of the benefit obligations incurred. Regular annual contributions build up the fund over the period of covered service. Another element which distinguishes private pensions from Social Security is that private benefits are directly related to the worker's salary and years of service, whereas Social Security benefits are to some degree related to salary and years of covered employment, but also involve considerable redistribution according to defined social objectives.

Perhaps the most precise definition of a private pension plan is that provided by the Employee Retirement Income Security Act of 1974 (ERISA):

> . . . any plan, fund, or program established or maintained by an employer or by an employee organization, or by both, that (a) provides retirement income to employees, or (b) results in a deferral of income by employees for periods extending to the termination of covered employment or beyond, regardless of the method of calculating the contributions made to the plan, the method of calculating the benefits under the plan or the method of distributing benefits from the plan (ERISA, Sec. 3(2)).

Since employers install pension plans, ERISA has also defined an employer:

> ... any individual, partnership, joint venture, corporation, mutual company, joint-stock company, trust, estate, unincorporated organization, association or employee organization acting directly as an employer or indirectly in the interest of an employer, in relation to an employee benefit plan (ERISA, Secs. 3(6) and 3(9)).

There were approximately 64 million employed persons in the private sector in 1974 (U.S. Department of Commerce, 1975). Of course, private organizations, partnerships, individuals, and so on, are not the only employers and not the only source of employee pension coverage. The number of federal government employees covered under the Federal Civil Service Retirement System was 2,665,600 in 1974 (U.S. Civil Service Commission, 1974). In addition, the armed services retirement plan covers approximately two million persons (U.S. Department of Commerce, 1976). Finally, state and local governments have nearly nine million full-time employees, most of whom belong to their employer's pension plan (U.S. Department of Commerce, 1976).

Private pension plans and public employee pension plans are usually discussed as separate entities. However the difference has more to do with the type of employer rather than with objectives or the type of pension plan, and from the standpoint of developing relevant public policy toward employee pension plans, it seems reasonable to suggest that public policy vis-à-vis both public and private employers should treat their pension plans as a single type, i.e., as employer-sponsored pension plans. This should enable legislative bodies and others to consider and develop regulatory approaches that provide for equal treatment of public and private employees under their pension coverage. Already, attention is being given to the question of whether public employee retirement systems should be brought under the recently enacted reform provisions that up to now cover only private plans. This and other questions are currently being considered by a Joint Pension Task Force under an ERISA mandate to study the implications of extending to public employers' plans the standards that were recently applied to private plans (ERISA, Sec. 3022a).

Background of Present Employee Retirement Plans. Our present system of employer-sponsored pensions (for both privately and publicly employed persons) originated in the latter part of the 19th century. But growth was slow, and it cannot be said that employee pension coverage—outside of a few industries and for teachers and police officers—became a significant factor in American economic and social life until the period of World War II.

The first pension plan in the private sector appears to have been that of the American Express Company, then a shipping company. However this was not, as is often assumed, a retirement plan as we now know such plans. It was a retirement *disability* plan: retirement under the plan was the consequence of disability rather than of old age as such, or of a mandatory retirement age. Thus under this plan only the disabled retired. Among plans for public employees, the earliest retirement arrangements were started in the 1870s, first for policemen and teachers. Here, too, disability was the normal condition for benefit eligibility.

The first large industry to exhibit interest in establishing employee pension plans was the railroads. In the closing years of the 19th century and the early years of the 20th, railroads saw the need for a way to ensure an orderly and socially acceptable way of retiring workers who were no longer able to meet the physical demands of their work because of age. Some other large industries too were beginning to have to face the problem of substantial numbers of employees reaching an age when work suffered, even though massive waves of immigrants helped to keep the national work force itself relatively young. Labor organizations also expressed growing interest in the economic security needs of their members, in addition to wage payments. At this time, however, labor was less interested in the area of retirement security than in the problems of survivors of members who died or became disabled. The relative youth of labor's membership helped focus its welfare interests primarily on workers' current needs.

In establishing their early pension plans, employers were generally unwilling to share control of the plans. There was no bargaining or labor-management coordination as we know it today. Nor were employers inclined to express pension commitments in terms that bound them for the future. Nearly all of the plans of this era described their benefits as gratuities granted at will, as revocable at any time, and as not constituting any binding future commitment.

By the end of 1929, as reported in Murray W. Latimer's (1932) pioneering study of industrial pension plans, 421 industrial pension plans had been established and 397 were still in operation. It was estimated that about 10 percent of the nonagricultural private work force was employed by the firms that had established pension plans, but by no means all of these employees were eligible for coverage, and only about 10 percent of those who were covered would actually receive any benefits, a situation largely attributable to the absence of vesting provisions on termination of employment. The coverage concentrated in the railroad industry and in such other industries as public utilities, iron and steel manufacturing, oil, banking, and general manufacturing (Bankers Trust Company, 1975). Latimer's study showed that pension plans in the private sector had developed mainly in the heavily capitalized, technologically advanced, and most rapidly growing industries. At the same time, a relatively high birth rate and continued immigration of men of working age kept high the ratio of young to old, and perhaps helps to explain the limited growth of pension plans in this period.

At the same time, public employee pension coverage had been growing slowly, especially in the 1920s, and by 1930 about a fourth of all state and local employees were employed by state and local units having plans. The Federal Civil Service Retirement System was started in 1920.

The Great Depression effectively slowed the growth rate of employee pension plans. But while private pensions faltered, old-age income support was put into an entirely new perspective by the creation in 1935 of the Social Security program, with taxes scheduled to start in 1937 and benefit payments to begin in 1941, later changed to 1940. This new social insurance program was generated by the shock of the depression and a vision of increasing numbers of elderly persons whose savings were lost and who would be without prospects for income support other than welfare. One of the issues at the time was whether the new social insurance program would stifle or even stop the growth of private pensions. Only later did it appear that it would function in part as a stimulus to the development of additional coverages.

In another important development of the depression, the federal government was forced to rescue the pension plans of the railroads, which found themselves with huge unfunded liabilities and no prospect of being able to pay for the promises they had made. The Railroad Retirement Act of 1935 effectively nationalized the railroads' pension plans, and can perhaps be regarded as a precursor (of sorts) of today's Pension Benefit Guaranty Corporation, since both were measures designed to protect and sustain private pension benefits through public intercession.

By 1940 about four million active workers were employees of companies administering retirement programs. Private plan assets and reserves in 1940 amounted to $2.4 billion (Bankers Trust Company, 1975). The Second World War brought a surge in the growth of coverage under private pension plans. Although wartime wage and price controls froze wages, additional compensation was permitted in the form of fringe benefits. Pension plans grew accordingly. Between 1940 and the end of the war in 1945, 2.5 million new workers became covered under private pension plans (Bankers Trust Company, 1975). Growth of coverage under public employee plans also continued to advance (U.S. Bureau of the Census, 1968).

Another important stimulus to the growth of private pension plans was a federal court decision later in the decade. In a 1948 dispute on whether pension plan coverage and benefits qualified as negotiable issues under labor contracts within the provisions of the Taft-Hartley Act, a federal court in the Inland Steel case held that pensions were negotiable items. This gave a considerable thrust to the development of new pension plans, and changed many existing pension plans from a matter of voluntary, unilateral action by employers into integral elements of the collective bargaining process (Inland Steel Co. *v.* NLRB, affirmed 170F.2nd 247 (C.C.A. 7, 1948)).

Between 1950 and 1970, the total number of active workers covered under pension plans in the private sector nearly tripled, reaching 26.1 million or about 45 percent of the private industrial labor force. In the same period, the number of recipients of private pensions rose more than tenfold, reflecting the gradual maturing of established plans. At the end of 1970, 4.7 million persons were receiving benefits from private pension plans. Total assets in 1970 reached $137 billion, and annual benefit payments $7.4 billion (Bankers Trust Company, 1975).

In government employment, the growth of pension coverage was even more impressive. The proportion of government employees participating in pension plans increased from about 50 percent following the end of World War II to over 90 percent in 1972 (U.S. Department of Commerce, 1954–1976).

Expressions of Public Policy. Public policy vis-à-vis private pensions has been expressed mainly through tax legislation. Until the mid-20s, private pensions developed and functioned without legislative hinderance or help. The Revenue Act of 1926 clarified a corporate income tax question by providing that pension plan earnings would not be taxed to a pension trustee or insurer. Until the early 1940s, this was the only governing federal legislation.

In 1942 a monumental new Internal Revenue Act was passed. This act contained the first substantive public policy considerations regarding the operation of private pension plans. It established conditions of pension plan "qualification" for the tax treatment of employer contributions to pension plans as a business expense, and for the continuation of the 1926 law dealing with the taxation of the investment earnings of pension funds. The major purpose of the "qualification" rules was to prevent the plans from discriminating in favor of officers, shareholders, supervisors, or highly compensated employees (Internal Revenue Code of 1954, Sec. 401a). The 1942 legislation also specified that employer contributions to a pension plan would not be taxed as current income to employees, but would be taxable to the employee when received as income. No vesting requirements were established; a Treasury recommendation that vesting standards be incorporated in the 1942 law was offered and then withdrawn (U.S. House Committee on Ways and Means, 1942).

The tax treatment of private pension plans established by the 1942 act (and by subsequent legislation) can be described as "favorable," in that it provided a few basic standards and some tax incentives to encourage the growth of pension protection.

However the 1942 legislation was limited in its scope. Until ERISA, the only additional significant federal acts of public policy regarding pension plans were limited to the Taft-Hartley Act (1947) and the Welfare and Pension Plans Disclosure Act (1958). The latter was designed to control financial abuses on the part of pension plan trustees, particularly among jointly administered and multiemployer plans in which serious breaches of fiduciary responsibility had been uncovered. As it turned out, reporting and disclosure requirements alone were insufficient means of correcting abuses (U.S. Code 1964, Title 29, Sec. 301 August 28, 1958).

The 1974 Pension Reform Act marked a new stage in public policy regarding private pension plans. The Congress in effect announced a new principle: private employers who make pension promises must follow extensive procedures that will assure their financial capacity to meet such promises. Furthermore, they must observe certain standards for vesting and eligibility under their plans, and they must disclose all plan provisions and conditions to employees participating in the plans and to the Treasury and Labor Departments. Although the ERISA legislation does not require that pension plans be provided by private employers, if plans are undertaken, public policy now requires that specific and extensive standards must be adhered to.

By the end of the year of the pension reform legislation, 1974 government statistics indicated that 29.8 million workers in the private sector were covered under a pension or profit-sharing plan (excluding Social Security). The figure is three times the coverage reported in 1950. The average annual rate of growth in coverage for the period 1950–1960 was 6.7 percent, for 1960–1970, 3.4 percent, and for 1970–1974, 3.4 percent. Table 1 summarizes the numbers of covered workers under private pension and profit-sharing plans by quinquennial years from 1950 to 1970, and annually thereafter through 1974.

The growth shown by Table 6.1 is encouraging, but for two reasons it is somewhat misleading. First, it must be noted that of the counted workers at any one time, not all of them will receive pension benefits in old age based on the pension plan under which they are counted as covered. This is because a covered worker is not necessarily a vested worker. Future benefits for nonvested workers are contingent on continuing plan membership until vesting requirements are met. If employment is terminated beforehand, the future benefits are forfeited. Second, although the number of covered workers has continued to grow, the growth rate of coverage as a percentage of the total private sector work force has been much slower in recent years. As Figure 1 shows, the work force has expanded at a rate faster than pension coverage.

In the public employee sector, the growth of employee pension coverage since 1945 has been nothing less than spectacular, both in the proportion of public employees covered and in the generosity of benefit promises (measured against the benefit formulas under private employers' plans). Between 1942 and 1967, the number of covered public employees increased from 1.5 to 7.1 million. Assets of state and local government employee pension plans grew from $1.865 billion in 1942 to $39.265 billion in 1967 (U.S. Bureau of the Census, 1968).

Status of Employee Pension Plans Today.   As we assess the potential of employee pension plans as income support systems for the elderly in the future, our starting point is the status of these plans as we begin the last quarter of the 20th century. Here, in brief, is what I believe should be taken into consideration as we plan for the future:

First, private pensions:

1. They are relatively young. Real growth did not begin until World War II.

Table 6.1   Covered Workers Under Private Pension and Deferred Profit-
           Sharing Plans, 1950–1974

Year	Number of Covered Workers (in thousands)
1950	9,800
1955	14,200
1960	18,700
1965	21,800
1970	26,100
1971	26,400
1972	27,500
1973	29,200
1974	29,800

Includes pay-as-you go, multiemployer, and union-administered plans, those of
nonprofit organizations, and railroad plans supplementing the Federal Railroad
Retirement Program. Excludes pension plans for Federal, State and local government employees as well as pension plans for the self-employed. Excludes beneficiaries.
Source: Skolnik (1976), p. 3, U.S. Department of Commerce (1954 through 1976).

2. Current figures suggest that the plans cover slightly less
    than half of the workers in the private sector.
3. The plans are concentrated among larger employers, in
    the more profitable industries, in the more heavily capital-
    ized industries, and in industries in which organized labor
    is strong.
4. The growth rate of private pension coverage as a propor-
    tion of the total private work force has slowed in recent
    years.

Figure 1 Covered Workers Under Private Pension and Profit-Sharing Plans[a] as a Percentage of all Employed Workers in the Private Sector, 1950–1974

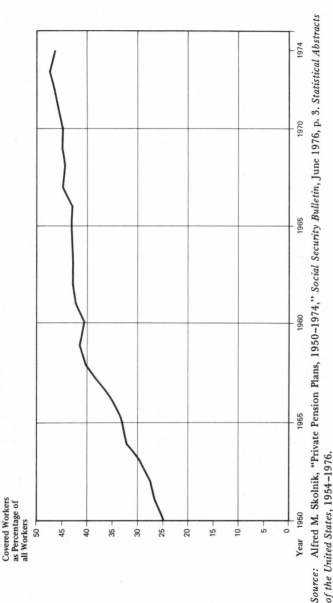

Covered Workers
as Percentage of
all Workers

Source: Alfred M. Skolnik, "Private Pension Plans, 1950–1974," *Social Security Bulletin,* June 1976, p. 3. *Statistical Abstracts of the United States,* 1954–1976.

[a] Includes pay-as-you-go, multiemployer, and union-administered plans, those of nonprofit organizations, and railroad plans supplementing the federal railroad retirement program. Excludes pension plans for federal, state, and local government employees and pension plans for the self-employed. Excludes beneficiaries.

5. Least likely to have pension coverage are employees in small firms, new firms, and industries in which labor organization is relatively weak. In some areas profit sharing or employee savings plans are a substitute for pensions.

6. So far, a relatively low proportion of workers who have been counted as "covered" under private pension plans at one time or another has actually received benefits from such plans when they retired. This is largely attributable to vesting delays that have been incorporated into pension plans. A 1972 Census Bureau study indicated that about one-third of the people covered by a private plan at the time of the survey had been vested under the plan (Kolodrubetz & Landay, 1973).

7. Private pension plans have varied greatly in their financial soundness. The requirements of ERISA will help gradually to reduce the unfunded liabilities of many plans and to assure the adequacy of current funding. The Pension Benefit Guaranty Corporation will mitigate the shock of termination of plans with unfunded liabilities, including young plans. The termination in 1964 of the Studebaker Corporation's pension plan was one of the events that focused attention on the need to back pension promises and pension coverage with the financial capacity to meet the obligations incurred. It is not so well known that the Studebaker Corporation's pension plan was only 13 years old, far younger than the corporation itself.

8. Virtually all employees in the private sector are covered under the Social Security system. Most plans provide for an integration of their benefits with those of the social insurance plan.

Contemporary public employee retirement plans exhibit some of the same characteristics as private plans, and differ in some respects:

1. The proportion of public employees covered under employer-sponsored pension plans is substantially higher than

the proportion of private employees. Over 90 percent of public employees, versus slightly less than half of private employees, enjoy membership in a pension plan.

2. Many public employee retirement systems are more seriously underfunded than private pension plans, and there is no Pension Reform Act to help engineer sounder financing. The problem of stranded beneficiaries on plan termination, however, does not appear to be as great as under private pension plans prior to ERISA, simply because governments seldom terminate. Nevertheless, knowingly to place future generations of taxpayers under the burden of huge unfunded pension liabilities, whether through neglect or intention, raises serious questions. The extent of the problem for future generations, who must ultimately face the cost, is illustrated by figures from just a few systems. The State University Retirement System of Illinois has reported for the year 1975 a funding deficiency of a half billion dollars (SURS Annual Report, 1975). The City of Los Angeles Fire and Police Pension System has liabilities of a billion dollars and assets of $200,000,000 (Patocka, 1973). In New York City the total underfunding of the city's pension funds is estimated at $6 billion; at this rate it would be necessary for the city to add $200 million to its budget annually for the next 30 years just to meet pension obligations already incurred (State of New York, 1976). Unfortunately, the extent of the unfunded pension liabilities of many public pension plans is usually not known by the public.

3. Many of the benefit formulas and funding methods of public employee pension plans were developed during a period when it appeared to some that there would be little or no limit to present or future tax revenues to support ever expanding promises and obligations. A favorable growth rate in real productivity in the private sector probably stimulated this attitude.

4. Benefit levels of public employee retirement systems are, on the average, higher than those in the private sector. Originally, differences were rationalized on the basis of the

lower pay scales of public employees. In recent years, however, the pay differentials have been eliminated and now
favor public employees.

5. As previously noted, there is no ERISA for public employee
retirement plans—no uniform requirements for funding
and fiduciary responsibility, or for vesting standards, or for
reporting and disclosure to participants.

6. Social Security coverage of state and municipal employees
is voluntary on the part of the employing unit. About two-
thirds of the members of public employee retirement systems are covered under the Social Security program.
Federal civil service employees are not covered under Social Security in the course of their federal employment, but
often gain it (in addition to a generous federal pension) in
other ways. In a number of states, Social Security was simply added on top of an existing state coverage without
integration, resulting in relatively high benefit replacement
ratios in comparison with private pensions, and in high
pension costs.

**Pension Plans and Future Demographic, Economic, and So-
cial Change.**   Reserve pension plans are less directly affected by
demographic changes than is the transfer system of Social Security. Although demographic changes affect private pensions
through their impact on the economy and their social consequences, this impact is cushioned by the fact that private pensions accumulate reserves for the purpose of meeting incurred
financial obligations for the specific groups covered. In the
longer term, changes in the birth rate will of course have many
economic and social results, which will influence the capacity of
employers to implement or revise benefit plans. Employment
patterns and profitability in specific sectors may also be affected,
but more generally. In all industries and geographic areas, demographic patterns sooner or later will affect employment patterns,
labor organizations, and markets, and all of these factors will
have an effect on the capacity of employers to inaugurate and
sustain employee pension plans.

Obviously, private and public employee pension plans cannot discharge their primary responsibility—the provision of retirement income—unless they are financially sound. A pension plan's good financial health depends on the provision of enough assets to meet incurred liabilities. This, in turn, depends upon the economic health of the organization providing the pension plan and on the health of that organization's industrial area and the American economy as a whole. Ultimately, every pension plan—public and private—rests on the national capacity for renewed capital formation, adequacy of investment return, productivity, and the continued capacity of the economy and the society to respond rationally and effectively to changing economic circumstances. Employee pension funds simultaneously depend upon and contribute to the capital formation process, which accumulates pension reserves to stand behind benefit payments promised for the future, and provides additions to capital as fuel for the economy. As a measure of the extent of this contribution, at the end of 1973 a total of $182.55 billion had been invested by private pension plans and $81.6 billion by state and local government employee pension plans. (Institute of Life Insurance, 1975). Over the next decade, it has been estimated that over $4.7 trillion will be required as new investment in order to sustain our economy at a reasonable growth rate (New York Stock Exchange, 1974). Pension plans are being relied upon more and more to provide the necessary lifeblood for the nation's economy (Drucker, 1975–1976).

If we are to say anything about the future of private pensions in social and economic terms, we must say that sound private pension plans require national economic policies that will enhance the process of savings and investment, encourage innovation and enterprise, and, while encouraging moderate growth, keep monetary inflation within reasonable bounds. It is perhaps no coincidence that the greatest growth of pension plan membership took place during the 1950s and early 1960s, years during which the average annual increase in the cost of living was about two percent, and years in which the gross national product grew from $533.5 billion (1950) to $925.9 billion (1965) (U.S. Department of Labor, 1975; U.S. Department of Commerce, 1976).

SOCIAL ATTITUDES. Pension plans are not only financial instruments, they are also instruments for the deferral of consumption. Thus pension plans involve the setting of priorities, and these priorities illustrate and determine what we do and are willing to do with respect to the comfort, health, and the income of the elderly. Under private and public employee pension plans, the express priority of income deferral takes the form of the setting aside of funds today to form the base of payments for tomorrow's retirement income. Under the Social Security program, the priority takes the form of the foregoing of current consumption by workers through the payment of the Social Security tax under an implied social contract that when the worker becomes eligible for the social insurance benefits, taxes paid by the next generation of workers will become the source of the benefit payments received. Under either the individual equity private pension systems or the social insurance system, the priority decision must be made, and it involves some degree of current sacrifice. Dr. Juanita Kreps has stated the priority propositions involved in the Social Security program clearly and eloquently:

> Thus, the current worker whose payroll is taxed to finance purchases made by current retirees is the provider in this stage of his life and the recipient in the next, and he is surely plagued with some obvious misgivings: how much of his own present earnings rightfully belong to today's retired worker? How will the amount he pays in OASDHI taxes compare with what he gets back when he retires? Will tomorrow's worker support him adequately? If not, what recourse will he have against the society, once he has ceased to be a productive worker? None of these questions is eased by the constant pressure on the worker's financial resources, which must cover ever-rising living costs, lengthened educational periods for his children, and frequently direct assistance to his own aged parents. . . .
>
> There are no simple solutions to the dilemma of today's worker. He could easily consume all his earnings, leaving no claims (either public or private) for future retirement needs. Social policy cannot hope to satisfy all his present and future needs, for they far outstrip his lifetime earnings. All social policy can do is provide a mechanism

that allocates aggregate output in some democratically agreed-to optimal fashion, the optimum allocation in this case having a lifetime as well as a temporary dimension. And just as there are differences of view as to how evenly income should be distributed at any point in time, so, too, men vary in the rates at which they discount the future—that is, in how highly they prize present over future consumption. . . .

. . . the particular mechanism we use for allocating income to the aged, i.e., the payroll tax paid into a social security "fund," directs attention to the tax burden borne by the worker on behalf of the retiree, and points up an apparent source of economic conflict between the two generations (U.S. Senate, 1970, p. 1924).

The recent White House Conference on Aging and the Older Americans' Act of 1965 have stated that retirement incomes for older persons should be "in accordance with the American standard of living." Such statements are useful, but to be realistic they must be accompanied by an understanding of the importance of setting priorities among competing limited resources, the need for the sound financing of the instruments used to provide retirement income, and the fact that the improvement of existing pension structures requires painful deferrals of current consumption. It is perhaps sobering to note that periods of retirement may approach in length almost half the length of a working lifetime, and that the building of pension reserves is thus a lifetime proposition if properly done.

ERISA.   Social considerations, public policy decisions on priorities, and our mode of going about the solution of long-range problems will determine the extent to which we introduce and support the costly and possibly disruptive actions that must be taken if planning for the future is to be adequate in the pension field. Despite its possible shortcomings, the Employee Retirement Income Security Act of 1974 (ERISA) stands as an example of action that builds on past accomplishments, recognizes the effectiveness of existing institutions (as well as their limitations), and builds for the long-term future. Implicit in ERISA is a recognition that in the past benefit promises were frequently made more freely than the capacity of the accompanying funding mechanisms warranted. ERISA recognizes that a sound private pension system needs public policy regulation to protect employees against loss of accrued benefits when vested rights have not been fully funded in a terminating plan. Employee pension plans needed the public policy support and direction that ERISA provided.

The provisions of ERISA occupy 240 pages of law and no doubt thousands of pages of regulations will ensue. The provisions are complicated. Nevertheless, this legislation is an honest effort to draft a law that would not overlook the many and often complex aspects of the process of assuring retirement income. ERISA's provisions perceive that the business of securing an income for life beginning at retirement involves many investment and administrative activities, requires institutional continuity and stability, and demands sound financial management and fiduciary conduct.

An early criticism of ERISA was that it resulted in waves of unexpected plan terminations, and that the legislation would in fact discourage the growth of pension planning (*New York Times,* 1976a). Other criticisms have been that ERISA's provisions are hopelessly complicated and that great additional employer expense is now being required to meet the new provisions, including both the funding provisions and the cost of reporting and disclosure.

When considering the criticism of increased plan terminations, it should be remembered that a substantial number of plans were terminated each year before the passage of ERISA. Also, reports of plan terminations sometimes do not include the balancing figures for new retirement plan approvals. In the first half of 1975, while 3,848 plan terminations were reported, 21,560 new plans were adopted (*Employee Benefit Plan Review,* 1975). A study of plan terminations in 1975 by the Pension Benefit Guaranty Corporation found that in over three-fourths of 4,300 terminations, ERISA requirements were not a factor, and that the most frequent causes of termination were adverse economic conditions during the year (*New York Times,* 1976b).

It is too early to come to firm conclusions about the effect of ERISA on pension plans, either in the short run or the long run. We must expect to hear a great deal about short-term dislocations, higher expenses, and confusing and inconsistent regulations. Reform legislation nearly always requires a period of adjustment. And new legislation often needs technical amendment; ERISA is no exception. Simplified reporting and elimination from the law of some of the "prohibited transactions" may well be among the first of the technical changes to be made. ERISA, however, has not just impeded or complicated pension plan operations, as some suggest. It codifies sound financial practice and plan provisions, establishing vesting and participation standards for the first time. The law opens the door to a greater future role for private pensions and should enhance the profile of old-age income, even though it will take time for those affected by the law to work their way through their plans to retired status and therefore into more favorable income statistics of the future.

The Future of Private and Public Employee Pensions. The development of institutions for private and public employee pension protection in the United States has been paralleled, more or less, by similar developments in the other Western industrialized nations. In each of these nations, private pensions are accompanied by a social insurance system to provide basic coverage as well as coverage for workers not associated with employer-sponsored plans for a sufficient length of time to become eligible for benefits. Our own recent reform legislation on the private pension side must await time for full assessment, but its effects should be positive.

With respect to the longer-range future of private pensions, several interlocking areas may be considered:

SOCIAL SECURITY. The relative role of the Social Security program in providing wage-related retirement income will affect the growth rate of private pensions. The early years of the Social Security program were characterized by relatively modest benefits. Those years were accompanied by a very rapid growth in the private pension sector. Now Social Security plays a larger part than it originally did in providing retirement income. In just the last six years, between 1971 and 1976, maximum retirement benefits under Social Security increased by 80 percent, or about 50 percent in constant dollars. But it does not seem likely that this rate of growth can continue, especially in light of the high future costs which even the present benefit promises will bring. Social Security is now a mature system, over 40 years old. It appears that through historical development and cost/benefit imperatives it has found its role as a base of benefits upon which other benefits can build. It seems unlikely that Congress will press for a larger role from Social Security as long as the present benefit levels themselves (including the CPI escalator feature) give evidence of requiring higher and higher payroll taxes in the future. This maturity suggests new opportunities for private pension and savings programs. Social Security transfer benefits, as a social base, can provide a third or more of the final year's pay for retiring workers with earnings histories of amounts below or up to the current Social Security wage base, and more for the retiree with an eligible spouse. With future adjustments for changes in living costs now incorporated into the program, it may be that employers and workers alike will turn greater attention to pension and profit-sharing plans as providers of supplementary retirement income.

RETIREMENT AGE. The question of what should be regarded as an appropriate retirement age is by no means settled, let alone whether there should be any mandatory age at all. Later retirement ages decrease the cost of a pension plan and increase the opportunity of workers to continue earning an income and to lead an active life. It seems almost certain that the future will bring a careful reexamination of retirement ages and of mandating retirement. Already it has been suggested that to control costs under the Social Security program, a future normal retirement age of 68, rather than 65, may be desirable. Many institutions of higher education have developed a flexible retirement age system, with normal retirement at age 65 but with extensions of service, on demonstration of continued capacity, to age 70. If, in the future, the question of the retirement date focuses more on individual capacities than on individuals as members of an age group, we may see more pension plans developing flexible retirement age policies. Or we may see the mandatory age of retirement rise—from 65 to 70, for example.

EARLY RETIREMENT PROVISIONS. In the last 10 years, many negotiated private pension plans have introduced "early and out" pension provisions. A number of public employee retirement systems provide for retirement with a full formula benefit when an employee completes a stated number of years of service, or meets a combined age and service requirement. And most pension plans have provisions for early retirement with actuarially reduced benefits. Recently, the U.S. Supreme Court decided that a state law mandating retirement for state police officers at an age below 65 does not violate the constitutional rights of employees so affected (Murgia *v.* Massachusetts Board of Retirement, 1976). The broader implications of this decision deserve careful analysis.

Although early retirement opens up opportunities for new uses of leisure time, recreation, and other personally-directed activities, it is also costly if the benefits are to be adequate. There is a shorter period over which to build up retirement income, and a longer period over which retirement benefits must be paid. In effect, early retirement is consumption now rather than later. An economic question for the future is whether American industry and workers can afford extensive early retirement provisions, which have the effect of reducing the work force as a percentage of the total population. Also to be considered are important social implications related to early retirement programs.

PENSION PORTABILITY. The question of pension portability, which received considerable discussion in the early stages of the development of ERISA legislation, has now come to be understood as largely a question of early vesting. From time to time, however, legislation is introduced into the Congress under the portability rubric designed to provide federal subsidies for state employees who move to another state and who have forfeited future benefits because they had not yet become vested in their retirement plan. But there is a better public policy answer to the lack of portability than federal subsidies for public employees who cross state lines. A fairer and more rational mode of improving portability would be to encourage earlier vesting in both public employee and private pension plans. Early vesting can help greatly in increasing the prospects for adequate pensions for people who change jobs frequently, whether it is within states or between them, or in public or private employment. A reasonable future public policy goal for all pension plans, public or private, should be a minimum requirement of 100 percent vesting on the completion of five years of service.

PUBLIC EMPLOYEE RETIREMENT SYSTEMS.   Overall, public employees have better pension protection than employees in the private sector, both in extent of coverage and benefit levels. In the future a primary need will be to formulate and implement practicable and proper funding standards for these plans in order to protect the rights of covered employees and at the same time to protect future taxpayers from inordinate financial burdens. In the next two decades, serious problems of overgenerous and underfunded public pension systems will face state and local governments as a result of the maturation of these plans and the swelling numbers of public employees that have entered the plans. It is to be expected that efforts to improve the funding of public employee pensions will, at least for the time being, slow the tendency of these types of plans to enlarge benefits far beyond those being received by retirees from the private sector, and will place public employee plans on a sounder financial footing. It is possible that Congress may attempt to devise legislation regarding funding standards of public employee retirement plans, although there are constitutional questions that remain to be worked out. Such legislation could be based on the public policies that have already been expressed for private pension plans in the 1974 Pension Reform Act.

UNPROTECTED PRIVATE WORKERS.   If one ultimate goal could be stated for private pension planning, no doubt it would be that every worker in the private sector, on retiring from employment, should receive a private pension or profit-sharing benefit along with Social Security. Yet, as we have seen, less than half of the private work force is employed by firms providing pension benefit plans. Therefore the next step to advance private pension protection must be through public policies that encourage employers and employees to set up pension plans where none exist today. Several possibilities have been suggested, and there are others. Employers without pension plans might, for example, be extended various types of favorable tax treatment if they agree to contribute matching amounts to an employee's Individual Retirement Account (IRA), the individual savings "substitute" for employer pension coverage that was added to the Internal Revenue Code (Section 219) by ERISA. IRAs currently provide a limited tax-deferred program for retirement savings for persons not participating in employer-sponsored pension plans. Another suggestion is that the amount of savings that may be put aside through tax deferral under the IRA program should be raised to the level of the Keogh Act (HR 10) plans, a mechanism for the provision of retirement income for self-employed professionals. Yet another suggestion is that employers without pension plans be taxed two percent of payroll, and that these funds be used by the government to establish substitute coverage for such employers' workers. Or employers might be mandated to provide modest levels of private pension coverage of the defined contribution type. Certainly the mechanisms available to small employers for the provision of pension protection should be as simple and inexpensive as possible.

PENSION GROWTH. It seems likely that pension plan coverage in the late 1970s will grow more slowly than in the early part of the decade. The more stringent provisions for employee participation required by ERISA may act to increase coverage within plans; on the other hand it is likely that new plans will be established at a lower rate, and already there have been some plan terminations by employers who cannot meet the funding standards of the new legislation. The next few years will be a period of transition for private pensions. During the 1980s, growth may resume if government policies encourage a climate of growth in the private sector as a whole, and if the economy is relatively healthy, with moderate rates of inflation and reduced unemployment.

Private pensions, public employee pensions, and the Social Security transfer system do not, of course, comprise our total system of income support for the elderly. It is a pluralistic system in keeping with other pluralistic aspects of our society. Income from paid work, income from the drawing down of personal assets or the yield on assets, assistance and gifts from relatives and friends, and welfare, comprise the total system. From a public policy standpoint, there seems little doubt that the most important elements of these sources that should be emphasized and strengthened are in the area of employer-sponsored pensions. Social Security benefit levels have grown greatly in past years, and the 1972 amendments further improved that system by introducing the automatic escalator related to the consumer price index. But the financial burden of the Social Security program now appears to be reaching its limit. Our opportunities now lie in the sectors of private and public employee pensions, and in trying to assure reasonable pension equity between those two areas of employment.

REFERENCES

Bankers Trust Company. *1975 study of corporate pension plans.* New York: Bankers Trust Co., 1975.

Drucker, P. Pension fund socialism. *The Public Interest,* 1975–1976, *46,* 3–46.

Employee Benefit Plan Review, October 1975, pp. 46, 48.

ERISA, Public Law 93-406, 29 U.S.C.

Institute of Life Insurance. *Statistical services,* 1975.

Kolodrubetz, W. W., & Landay, D. M. Coverage and vesting of full-time employees under private retirement plans. *Social Security Bulletin,* 1973, *36,* 27.

Latimer, M. W. *Industrial pension systems in the United States and Canada, 1.* New York: Industrial Relations Counselors, Inc., 1932.

New York Stock Exchange. *The capital needs and savings potential of the U.S. economy.* New York: New York Stock Exchange, 1974.

New York Times, March 8, 1976a.

New York Times, March 21, 1976b.

Patocka, B. Public funds: The Herculean task is underway. *Pensions,* 1973, *2*(2), 33–48.

Skolnik, A. M. Private Pension Plans, 1950–1974. *Social Security Bulletin,* 1976, *39*(6), 3–17.

State of New York, Executive Department, Permanent Commission on Public Employee Pension and Retirement Systems, Report. *Recom-*

mendation for a new pension plan for public employees: The 1976 coordinated escalator retirement plan. March 1976.

SURS Annual Report. State University Retirement System of Illinois, 1975.

U.S. Bureau of the Census. Census of governments, 1967, 6(2). Employee-Retirement Systems of State and Local Governments. Washington, D.C.: U.S. Government Printing Office, 1968.

U.S. Civil Service Commission, Bureau of Retirement, Insurance, and Occupational Health. Annual report of financial and statistical data for fiscal year ended June 30, 1974. Washington, D.C.: U.S. Government Printing Office, 1974.

U.S. Department of Commerce, Bureau of the Census. Statistical abstract of the United States. Washington, D.C.: U.S. Government Printing Office, 1954–1976.

U.S. Department of Commerce. Survey of Current Business, 1976, No. 1, Part 11.

U.S. Department of Labor. Monthly Labor Review, 98(11), 1975.

U.S. House of Representatives, Committee on Ways and Means, Hearings, Revenue Revisions of 1942. 77th Cong., 2nd Sess. Memorandum submitted by Randolph E. Paul (March 23, 1942), pp. 1004–1005. Washington, D.C.: U.S. Government Printing Office, 1942.

U.S. Senate, Special Committee on Aging. Economics of aging: Toward a full share in abundance, Hearings. 91st Cong., 2nd Sess., May 4, 5, and 6, 1970. Prepared statement by Dr. Juanita Kreps.

-Part IV-

INCOME-IN-KIND

The previous two sections of this book have been devoted to the cash income of the elderly. The three chapters in this section—on U.S. health care, European health-related care, and U.S. social services—cover some of the considerations of affecting future policy options for provision of income-in-kind.

According to Henry Brehm, the major U.S. health care objective over the next quarter century will be the reshaping of the delivery system and simultaneous control of the inflation of costs. Brehm is optimistic about the effects of cost control: if executed properly, he argues, it could actually promote better care, by reducing hospitalization and encouraging the use of extended care facilities, outpatient ambulatory and day bed services, and home health care. Moreover, controlling costs should further the fortunes of health maintenance organizations, which Brehm argues are very good providers of care. The focus of Brehm's paper is very much on the issue of costs; policy issues such as how to provide better integration of social and health care systems are not explored.

Esther Ammundsen's paper, which follows, offers a glimpse of the kinds of problems which the U.S. might face in the future. Most European countries are relatively advanced in providing health and social services. They have adopted a number of different methods to integrate these services and are utilizing a variety of models of centralization and decentralization of control. Serious problems persist, however, particularly in the over-utilization of institutional care. Moreover, provision of primary care by general practitioners has been allowed to deteriorate in many instances, and the need for preventive care has not been met. Europe is farther ahead than the U.S., but is still looking for answers.

American experts have done a good deal of thinking about what kind of at-home services can reduce unnecessary institutionalization, but relatively little analysis of how to integrate them into an effective health care system. Existing at-home services are provided under a variety of auspices, including local health departments and departments of social welfare. A few are provided under the Older Americans Act. However these account for only a small fraction of public dollars expended on income-in-kind for older people. In 1975, for example, the whole Older Americans

Act was budgeted at only $552 million, compared to the over $14 billion spent on Medicare alone. Despite the act's limited scope, a chapter on it has been included because the Area Agencies for which it provides have generated high expectations, and seem to be contenders for the role of coordinators of integrated services.

As director of a state agency on aging, Robert Benedict provides an insider's look at the problems and prospects of Older Americans Act programs. The major and most immediate problem, as he sees it, is the enormous gap between the expectations raised by the Area Agencies and their limited capacity to fulfill these expectations—a gap which he believes may threaten the agencies' existence. His proposed solutions reflect his strong belief that the act can make a valuable contribution. For instance, he suggests shifting focus from planning to providing service and quadrupling the number of Area Agencies; decentralizing program administration and establishing local accountability; and training many new professionals.

Because the elderly of the future will be increasingly well educated, vigorous, and involved, Benedict suggests the act's focus could be narrowed to the single mission of serving the functionally disabled aged. Although he does not make a major point of this suggestion, it is a far-reaching recommendation, underscoring the Federal Council on the Elderly's concern with the frail elderly, and moving away from treating all people over 65 as a distinct class. Such a shift would allow the Area Agencies to take on new functions, such as becoming long-term care management organizations.

It is not within the scope of this book to provide equal time for those proposing alternate ways of integrating health and social services. Nonetheless, such integration is a key issue affecting the well-being of the future elderly. Its relative neglect by those planning our national health insurance program needs to be remedied soon, because the lack of integration is a problem that will not vanish even if we succeed in our current objective of clamping controls on health care costs. And, as Esther Ammundsen has observed of the various European arrangements, once systems are in place, they are hard to change.

-7-

The Future of U.S. Health Care Delivery for the Elderly

Henry P. Brehm

In attempting to discuss what changes are likely to occur over the next 10 to 25 years in the delivery and use of health-related services for the elderly, certain assumptions have to be accepted. First, we must assume that there will be a continuing national commitment to the concept of the right to health and health care unimpeded by personal financial resources.

Second, prediction and forecasting are reasonable exercises only if they are based on observable trends or known or anticipated factors. Under this assumption, we can discuss the potential future impact of expected demographic changes, of certain proposed changes in the organization and financing of health care, and of extrapolating trends in utilization patterns and other related social and economic factors. We cannot anticipate what scientific or medical breakthroughs may be made in the content of care.

We will start with an assessment of the expected changes in the size and percentage of the aged population in this country, compared to changes that have occurred in the recent past. Then the relevant issues to be considered center on trends in health care use over time; differences in amount and patterns of use between age groups; potential need for more facilities used primarily by the aged and brought on by projected population changes; and factors in the organization and financing of health care in general and for the aged in particular which may affect use and cost.

To deal with these items it will be necessary (1) to analyze the use of various types and levels of care as well as trends in this use by the aged as compared to other segments of the population; (2) to assess the impact which existing programs such as Medicare and Medicaid have had on this use; (3) to consider the potential impact of financing programs such as national health insurance on overall utilization as well as on utilization among the aged; and (4) to discuss the present trends in medical care organization and financing as they might be expected to influence total use and the patterns of use of services and facilities.

Within this context, we can then speculate on changes that might be expected in the delivery of health-related services, and make some assessment of the relative importance of various factors and pressures on these anticipated changes.

DEMOGRAPHIC INFLUENCES

What demographic changes can we expect in the next 25 years which might influence the delivery of health care to the elderly? The U.S. Bureau of the Census in October 1975 issued *Population Estimates and Projections* which uses three different sets of fertility assumptions to estimate both the total population of the U.S. and its age distribution. Table 7.1–7.3 summarize these data.

The U.S. had a more dramatic rate of increase in its aged population from 1950 to 1975 than is projected for the period between 1975 and 2000 under any of the Census Bureau's series of assumptions about future population trends. As a percentage of the population, the aged comprised 8.1 percent in 1950 and 10.5 percent in 1975. This will probably rise to 11.7 percent in the year 2000, is Series II (Table 7.2) is taken as the best estimate. (Series I and III are the result of applying a 10 percent correction factor above and below the cohort fertility assumptions used for Series II.) The data indicate that there has been a greater change in the proportion of the population which is aged in the 1950–

Table 7.1 U.S. Population Age 65 and Over: Projections from Years 1975–2000 by Age Subgroups (in Thousands)

Age	1975 No.	%	1980 No.	%	1985 No.	%	2000 No.	%
65+	22,330	100.0	24,523	100.0	26,659	100.0	30,600	100.0
65 – 74	13,881	62.2	15,412	62.8	16,389	61.5	17,079	55.8
75 – 84	6,627	29.7	7,041	28.7	8,005	30.0	10,304	33.7
85+	1,822	8.2	2,071	8.4	2,265	8.5	3,217	10.5

Source: U.S. Department of Commerce (1975).

Table 7.2   U.S. Population Age 65 and Over: Projections from Years 1975–2000 by Subgroups

As percent of total U.S. population--by projection series

	1975	1980 Series			1985 Series			2000 Series		
		I	II	III	I	II	III	I	II	III
65+	10.5	10.9	11.0	11.1	11.0	11.4	11.7	10.7	11.7	12.5
65 – 74	6.5	6.8	6.9	7.0	6.8	7.0	7.2	6.0	6.5	7.0
75 – 84	3.1	3.1	3.2	3.2	3.3	3.4	3.5	3.6	3.9	4.2
85+	0.9	0.9	0.9	0.9	0.9	1.0	1.0	1.1	1.2	1.3

Source: U.S. Department of Commerce (1975).

Table 7.3 Change in U.S. Population Age 65 and Over: Projections from Years 1975–2000 by Age Subgroups

<u>Percent change in population category</u>

	<u>1950-1975[a]</u>	<u>1975-1980[b]</u>	<u>1975-1985[b]</u>	<u>1975-2000[b]</u>
Total population	+40.3	+4.4	+9.7	+23.0
65+	+80.1	+9.8	+19.4	+37.0
65 - 74	+64.6	+11.0	+18.1	+23.0
75 - 84	+118.8[c]	+6.2	+20.8	+55.5
85+		+13.4	+24.3	+76.6

[a] 1950 population was used as the base for percent.
[b] 1975 was used as the base for percent.
[c] Percent change is for age 75+.
Source: U.S. Department of Commerce (1970, Table 24, and 1975, Table 1).

1975 period than is projected in the next 25 years. The rate of change in the size of the population 65 and over was also more dramatic from 1950 to 1975, when it showed an 80 percent increase, than from 1975 to 2000, when it is projected, under all assumptions, to increase by 37 percent. In evaluating these data it must be remembered that as subsequent base years become larger, a constant increase in numerical size will result in a decreased rate of increase. However, when we look at the increases in absolute numbers of aged persons, we see a larger increase from 1950 to 1975 than from 1975 to 2000. The last 25 years have seen an increment of approximately two million every five years. Approximately the same magnitude of increase will be maintained until 1990, when it will drop and remain at a lower magnitude of increase until after 2005. Then it will substantially increase again as a result of different size birth cohorts beginning in 1940.

Even with these increases in the numbers of aged persons, their proportion in the population is projected to be only nominally larger by the year 2000 because of the anticipated growth in the total population. Thus, while the numbers of aged persons will grow by 37 percent from 1975 to 2000, the total population will grow by 23 percent. From 1950 to 1975 the comparable rates of increase were 80 percent and 40 percent.

The age distribution within the 65-plus age group is expected to shift between now and the year 2000. The population 75 and over will grow at a faster rate than the population aged 65–74. In 1975, 4 percent of the total U.S. population was 75 and over; in 2000 the projected rate is 5.1 percent. Within the 65-plus population 37.9 percent were 75 and over in 1975; by 2000 this figure will grow to 44.2 percent. The absolute numbers of people aged 75–84 will grow by 55.5 percent by the year 2000; the 85 and over group will grow 76.6 percent. The population aged 75 and over grew by the much higher rate of 119 percent from 1950 to 1975.

These data point to a definite increase in the number and proportion of elderly persons in the U.S. population over the next 25 years. However the data show that the rate of change will be less abrupt than it has been in the past 25 years. The U.S. population will add more elderly persons between now and the year 2000, but the rate of increase will be lower than has been true since 1950. It is the population aged 75 and over that is projected to show the most dramatic increase relative to its present size. However this will result in an increased proportion of just over one percent of the total population (4% to 5.1%) in a period of 25 years. The increase is only sizable relative to the present absolute number of persons in that age group.

Potential Impact of Demographic Changes on Health Care Delivery. Will this increase in the population aged 65 and over, or in subparts of that population require or produce any changes in health-related services in the near or middle-range future? Such a question cannot be considered solely from the perspective of the projected population changes. This is especially the case given the data presented on past, relative to anticipated, population changes. That the delivery and financing of medical care in the U.S. will undergo change is beyond dispute. It has undergone change in the past 25 years. In some ways this change has been quite dramatic. However, will the population changes require extreme measures? Is projected population change the most significant factor to be faced by the medical care delivery system in the changes it will probably undergo and the changes that can be recommended for it over the next 25 years? A review of such issues is intricately tied in with the nature of health care and health care delivery and financing.

Unlike some areas of social program and service delivery, health services are not needed or used exclusively by the aged, nor are they primarily oriented toward meeting the demands of the aged. All age segments of the population make demands on the health care delivery resources of this country, albeit in differing amounts and with differing requirements. On the other hand, public income maintenance programs traditionally are oriented primarily toward support of the aged and dependent children, with special exceptions for those young and middle-aged adults who are considered unable to work. Changes in the ratio between working-age persons and the aged and changes in the overall dependency ratio are critical for assessing the potential burden of such support to be borne by each working-age person. However the provision and use of medical care services is a somewhat different situation. In this area the issue is the differential rates of use and patterns of use by different age groups, and the impact that changes in the age distribution will have an overall utilization of specific services and facilities.

If programs such as Medicare and Medicaid were the only ones concerning us, then dependency ratios would be a significant issue in assessing the burden for the public financing of medical care for the aged. However we anticipate the passage of some form of national health insurance before the end of the century. Current debates have centered more on specifics than on the principle of whether responsibility for the financing of health care should be borne by the population at large through government involvement. Under these circumstances, resources allocated for the public financing of health care use by the aged as compared to other age groups is proportional to the relative use and cost of health care by different age groups. The working-age population will bear the major burden for financing all care paid for with public funds. Costs for the health care of the elderly will increase this burden to the extent that their costs become a higher percentage of the cost of all health care, and/or to the extent that an increased percentage of the gross national product is devoted to health care.

TRENDS IN USE AND COST OF HEALTH SERVICES

In reviewing the use of health services by the aged, we will focus on the change over time in patterns of use. Use of relative to other age groups will serve as a basis for comparison.

Physician Visits. As Table 7.4 shows, physician visits per person per year for all age groups was 5.0 in 1973. For those 65 and over the rate was 6.5 For those over 45, the differences between age groups in the number of physician visits have, if

Table 7.4 Number of Physician Visits per year, 1963–1973

Age:	July 1963–June 1964	July 1966–June 1967	1969	1971	1973
All persons	4.5	4.3	4.3	4.9	5.0
Under 5 years	5.5	5.7	5.7	6.8	6.5
5 – 14	2.8	2.7	2.8	3.3	3.4
15 – 24	4.3	4.0	3.7	4.5	4.5
25 – 34	4.7	4.4	4.4	5.1	5.3
35 – 44	4.4	4.3	4.1	4.5	4.9
45 – 54	4.8	4.3	4.3	5.1	5.4
55 – 64	5.3	5.1	5.1	5.9	5.5
65 – 74	6.3	6.0	6.1	6.4	6.5
75 and over	7.3	6.0	6.2	7.2	6.6

Source: National Center for Health Statistics (1975, Table B).

anything, become smaller since 1963. For the total population there has been an increase in average visits per year since 1966–1967, after a small drop from 1963–1964 to 1966–1967. For those 65–74 the pattern is more stable and shows a smaller increase. For those 75 and over there is an irregular pattern which does not show a net increase over the decade.

The fact is that use by age groups under 65 has been increasing more than use by those 65 and over. Therefore it is unlikely that the projected increase in the proportion of the population which is over 65 will mean that older people's share of physician use will increase in the next 25 years.

Hospital Care. In the use of hospital services, there are more pronounced differences among age groups and over time. The rate of admission to general and special hospitals per 1,000 persons in the total population increased from 110 in 1950 to 146 in 1965 (the last full year before the Medicare amendments to the Social Security Act went into effect) and to 148 in 1967.

In 1963, well before the passage of Medicare, the rate of admission to short-term hospitals was 180 per 1,000 person-years for those 65 and over, compared to 130 per 1,000 person-years for the total population. With the exception of the increased hospital admission rate for the child-bearing years, there was a definite trend of increased hospital use with age.

For the population 65 and over, the rate of admission to short-term general hospitals was 275 per 1,000 population in 1967, rising to 314 per 1,000 in 1971. For the Medicare-enrolled population, the trends are quite consistent. In 1969 the hospital admission rate was 307 per 1,000 enrollees. This rose to 320 per 1,000 in 1973.

Two trends are evident in these data. There is a higher rate of hospitalization for those age 65 and over than for younger members of society; and the hospital admission rate for those 65 and over has grown substantially over the years, particularly from before to after the introduction of Medicare.

At the same time that hospital admission rates for the aged have been increasing, average lengths of stay have been generally

Table 7.5   Admission Rates per 1000 Total Population and Average Length of Stay, General and Special Hospitals, 1950–1967

	1950	1955	1960	1965	1966	1967
Admission Rate	110	125	136	146	146	148
Average length of stay:						
in days	10.6	9.9	9.3	9.1	9.5	9.1

Source: U.S. Department of Commerce (1969).

Table 7.6 Hospital Admissions per 100 Person-Years, 1963

	All Ages	Ages				
		0-5	6-17	18-34	35-54	55-65	65 and over
Admission rate	13	8	6	19	14	17	18

Source: Andersen and Anderson (1967), reprinted with the permission of The University of Chicago Press.

Table 7.7 Short-Term General Hospital Utilization, Persons Aged 65 and Over

	1967	1968	1969	1970	1971
Admission rate per 1000 aged persons	275	285	301	310	314
Average length of stay (days)	12.7	13.3	13.2	12.8	12.4

Source: West (1971).

Table 7.8 All Hospital Inpatient Admissions, Hospital Insurance Enrollees Under Medicare

	1969	1970	1971	1972	1973
Admission rate per 1,000 HI enrollees	307	307	305	313	320
Average length of covered stay (days)	-	13.1	12.6	12.1	11.7

Source: U.S. Department of Health, Education, and Welfare (1976b).

decreasing after an upswing in average length of stay during the first few years after Medicare went into effect.

In Karen Davis's 1975 analysis of the distribution of Medicare benefits by socioeconomic characteristics, she notes that after the advent of Medicare there was a decrease in the disparity between the hospitalization rate of blacks compared to that of whites. The implication is that (at least in this one area of medical care) the reduction of a financial barrier to care altered the pattern of use for a group which has traditionally had lower levels of utilization. In the data Davis presents (Table 7.9), it is apparent not only that there was a differential rate of change between the races in the use of hospitalization before and after Medicare, but that there was a pronounced difference in the rate of persons hospitalized per 1,000 population (as distinct from admission rate) by age groups. For those under 65, the pre-to-post Medicare rate of persons hospitalized shows a decrease after Medicare. For those 65 and over, regardless of race, there is a substantial increase.

These presumed effects of Medicare demonstrate the degree to which patterns and trends in medical care use may be alterable based on a change in the financing system available.

Nursing and Personal Care Homes. Nursing and personal care homes are a special category of health-related facility used almost exclusively by the elderly. In 1963 there were 505,242 residents in nursing and personal care homes in the United States. Of these, 11.8 percent were under age 65 (Table 7.10), whereas 70.4 percent were 75 and over. The number of residents per 1,000 population was 0.6 for the population under 65, 57.1 for those 75 and over, and 148.4 for those 85 and over (Table 7.11). By 1969, after the Medicare and Medicaid programs were well into operation, the age distribution of residents in nursing and personal care homes was not much different from what it had been in 1963, but the number of residents per 1,000 population was quite dramatically higher, particularly among the very old. It was still only 0.5 per 1,000 population for those under 65, but had increased to 76.6 per 1,000 population for those 75 and over. The residents per 1,000 population aged 65–74 had gone up from 7.9 in 1963 to 11.1 in 1969. The number of residents in

Table 7.9 Persons Hospitalized per 1000 Population, by Race and Age, Selected Years

	White	Black and other races
All ages		
1961-1962	95	73
1966	103	81
1968	97	83
Under age 15		
1961-1962	52	36
1966	58	43
1968	46	39
Age 15 - 44		
1961-1962	125	114
1966	125	120
1968	113	116
Age 45 - 64		
1961-1962	98	68
1966	112	83
1968	102	90
Age 65 and over		
1961-1962	114	78
1966	134	88
1968	158	126

Source: Davis (1975), reprinted with the permission of the Milbank Memorial Fund Quarterly.

nursing and personal care homes increased from 309,858 to 815,100 residents.

In absolute numbers, the population of these homes had grown by 227,755 persons who were 75 and over. If we apply the 1963 rates of residents per 1,000 population to the 1969 population for the 75–84 and 85-plus age groups, the growth in the nursing home population would have been only 81,932. The remainder of this increase is based on a change in pattern of use and not on an increase in the size of the very old population. If

Table 7.10 Number and Percentage Distribution of Residents in Nursing and Personal Care Homes, by Age

	1963		1969	
	Number	Percent	Number	Percent
Total	505,242	100.0	815,100	100.0
Age				
Under 65	59,678	11.8	92,900	11.4
65 - 74	89,619	17.7	138,500	17.0
75 - 84	207,243	41.0	321,800	39.5
85+	148,702	29.4	261,900	32.1

Source: National Center for Health Statistics (1965; 1973).

241

Table 7.11   Number of Residents in Nursing and Personal Care Homes
             per 1000 Population by Age

	1963	1969
All ages - 20+	4.5	4.0[a]
20 - 64	0.6	0.5[a]
65 - 74	7.9	11.1
75+	57.1	76.6
75 - 84	39.6	[b]
85 and over	148.4	[b]

[a]For 1969, these rates are based on the entire population of concern and do not exclude those under 20.
[b]Data not available for 1969.
Source: National Center for Health Statistics (1965; 1973).

we apply the 1969 rates to the projected 65-plus populations of the years 1985 and 2000, we will need space for an additional 246,400 elderly persons in nursing and personal care homes in 1985, and for an additional 503,086 in the year 2000. This annual rate of increase in residents from 1969 through those years would be slower than the rate from 1963 to 1969. Accommodating such an increase should be no more difficult than accommodating the change from 1963 to 1969, whether by increasing capacity use or by building to increase the capacity.

If the rate of residents to 1,000 population increases as dramatically in the next 25 years as it did from 1963 to 1969, an entirely different situation will be created. However the 1963–1969 increase in the number of very old people in nursing and personal care homes was not primarily the result of a higher number of elderly people in our society, but of an increase in their rate of use of these homes. Such a pattern and its trend of change over time is a factor of the medical care delivery system which is not the result of population changes, and is therefore potentially controllable if there is a desire to exercise control over the delivery system, its use, and the economic resources devoted to it.

Cost of Health Care. These patterns and trends in the use of physicians, hospitals, and nursing and personal care homes are based on rates, and they are therefore independent of changes in the size of the aged population. However, in combination with inflation rates, they have significantly affected the overall and the per capita levels of expenditures for health care and the percentage of the gross national product used for health-related goods and services over the last several years.

Tables 7.12 and 7.13 provide data on national health expenditures and the changes that have taken place since 1950. The total national health expenditure in fiscal year 1950 was $12,028 million, which amounted to 4.6 percent of the gross national product. Preliminary estimates for fiscal year 1974 show a total expenditure of $104,239 million, or 7.7 percent of the gross national product. The per capita expenditure rose in the same time period from $78.35 to $485.36. If we apply the 1950 per capita figure to the 1974 population, there would have been an increased total expenditure not of $92 billion, but of $4.8 billion. In other words, slightly over five percent of the total increase in expenditure can be attributed to population growth, the rest being the result of inflation in unit costs and increases in levels of utilization.

The major specific items of increase in per capita health expenditure from 1950 to 1974 were hospital care, which went from $24.09 to $190.44, and nursing-home care, which went from $1.16 to $34.69.

When we look at the change in per capita costs for personal health care for the elderly from just prior to Medicare to several years after Medicare, we see a pattern of continuous year-by-year increase of approximately $100 per capita—from $445 in fiscal 1966 to $1,218 in fiscal 1974. Again, hospital and nursing home care showed the steepest rates of increase, from $177.84 and $68.39 in 1966 to $573.18 and $289.10, respectively, in 1974.

Table 7.12   National Health Expenditures for Fiscal Years 1950 and 1974

	1950	1974
Aggregate amount (millions)	$12,028	$104,239
Per capita aggregate expenditure	$78.35	$485.36
Aggregate as percentage of GNP	4.6	7.7
Per capita hospital care	$24.09	$190.44
Per capita physicians services	$17.52	$88.47
Nursing-home care	$1.16	$34.69

Source: U.S. Department of Health, Education and Welfare (1976a)

These data on use and cost of health services indicate that the increases in demand and expenditures for such services over the past 10 to 25 years have primarily been the result of changes in patterns of use of these services and in dramatic increases in their cost. These changes occurred during a period when the absolute numbers and relative proportions of the aged increased at a more dramatic rate than is projected over the next 25 years. Some, but by no means all of these increases were unquestionably related to the advent of Medicare and Medicaid. The history of increases in the levels of use and the percentages of the gross national product as well as per capita expenditures devoted to health care attest to this fact.

Given this record of changes in use and cost of health-related services over the last several years, it is probable that our ability to rationalize the use of services and to exercise some control over their delivery and their financing will be more significant than changes in the elderly population itself.

What efforts have we made to influence the way in which health services are delivered or financed? The most important legislation was the 1965 amendments to the Social Security Act which authorized Medicare and Medicaid.

Impact of Medicare on Health Care for the Elderly. We have already reviewed some of the data indicating the changes that took place in the use and cost of medical care for the elderly from before to after Medicare went into effect.

Aside from these indications of the impact of Medicare on the use and cost of care for the aged, there are other data available which document its effect on the system for delivery of care. In a study of the health delivery system in Kansas City (Coe, Brehm & Peterson, 1974) which compared the situations just before and two and four years after the advent of Medicare, no appreciable change was noted in the organization of health care services. Although they recognized the need for other levels of care, most physicians had not altered their methods of practice. Few plans made to expand facilities and services just after Medicare was implemented were actually carried out, and no further Medicare-

Table 7.13 Estimated Per Capita Personal Health Care Expenditures for Population 65 and Over, 1966–1974.

Year	Hospital care	Physicians' services	Nursing-home care	Total
1966	$177.84	$ 89.57	$ 68.39	$445.25
1967	223.58	108.97	84.94	535.03
1968	282.89	122.40	113.56	646.65
1969	335.76	127.49	133.18	735.19
1970	375.13	141.60	162.76	828.31
1971	418.55	154.37	202.39	925.98
1972	468.61	172.58	237.79	1033.51
1973	508.93	180.74	265.11	1119.78
1974	573.18	182.14	289.10	1217.84

Source: U.S. Department of Health, Education, and Welfare (1976a).

related change in services was contemplated. There was no coordination between nursing homes and hospitals.

These findings ran counter to the implicit, if not the explicit intent of Medicare, which was to affect the provision, organization, and patterns of referral for health services for the aged within a community's health care subsystem. It was expected that Medicare would result in an expansion and coordination of facilities and services so as to provide more comprehensive services for the elderly, including transitional forms of inpatient care (extended care facilities) and ambulatory care services. The referral pattern among providers was also expected to change and expand to enable continuity among various types and levels of care.

In the study cited earlier, Davis draws the following conclusion:

> The major conclusion of the study is that a uniform medical care financing plan has not been sufficient to guarantee equal access to medical care for all elderly persons. Those elderly population groups with the poorest health are the lowest utilizers of medical care services under the program—the poor, blacks, and residents of the South. Furthermore, differences on the basis of income, race, and location are of sizeable magnitude (p. 480).

She goes on to note that "the structure of the Medicare program, through its reliance on uniform cost-sharing provisions for all elderly persons, is largely responsible for the greater use of medical services by higher income persons." Davis makes the following recommendations:

> Several changes in the Medicare program are required to reduce the inequities revealed by the current distribution of benefits. Four areas which seem particularly in need of reexamination are (1) the cost-sharing structure of Medicare, (2) efforts to improve access of minorities to medical care, (3) the sources of financing for Medicare, and (4) the method of physician reimbursement (p. 481).

Against this background of the impact of Medicare and recommendations for its alteration, we need to look to what possible approaches might be taken for health care in general, and for health services for the aged in particular. Another concern is how we might best get where we want to go.

ORGANIZATION AND FINANCING OF THE HEALTH CARE DELIVERY SYSTEM

The general direction in which we should be heading was suggested by Coe and Brehm (1972) in the concluding section of their book, *Preventive Health Care for Adults.*

> Since a considerable amount of research has shown time and again that our present fee-for-service organization of medicine is dysfunctional in terms of providing certain groups with adequate medical care—especially the poor and the aged—it would seem reasonable that some form of subsidized care would be provided. Medicare and Medicaid, of course, already provide some precedent for this approach. But these programs are not oriented to altering the present system for delivery of medical care. They provide financial support for the present system of delivery which is oriented primarily toward dealing with illness, not promoting health. What is needed is a combination of subsidized care and a reorientation of the delivery system to a coordinated comprehensive system concerned with the maintenance of a maximum health condition and preventing, as well as dealing with illness. Such a reorientation coupled with a reorganization of the delivery system would incorporate the physician into an organizational network which coordinates his efforts with those of other medical and paramedical specialists. This would relieve the doctor of the need to spend his time performing tests and other functions which can be handled by specialists and technicians with lesser levels of training. It would also alter the existing concepts of needed physician/patient ratios thereby easing some of the upward pressure on the cost of medical care and partially relieving the shortage of fully trained physicians (pp. 124–125).

How we arrive at this position involves both planning and promotional efforts, as well as experimentation with various delivery organizations and financing mechanisms. Among the devices being considered and actively pursued are some form of national health insurance, wider availability of health maintenance organizations (HMOs), and increased use of physician extenders, nurse practitioners, etc.

National Health Insurance. Given the many sponsors for legislation proposing national health insurance, it seems reasonable to expect that the United States will ultimately adopt such a measure for the financing of care. However it is also highly probable that our first national health insurance program will be restricted to providing a mechanism to finance the use of health care on a cost-sharing basis, with part of the cost of care paid by the user, and part by the government or other insurer.

HMOs. At the level of organization for delivery, the recognized need to provide more coordinated, comprehensive health care services and at the same time to contain the rapid increase in health care costs has given rise to a series of planning and experimenting techniques. The HMO Act of 1973 and the inclusion of HMOs under the Medicare reimbursement program are two mechanisms to encourage this prepaid group practice arrangement as a potentially more effective and cost-conscious approach to delivery.

Although these mechanisms are designed to promote HMOs, there is concern that some of the requirements placed on them to qualify for federal funds may restrict their competitive position. At the same time, efforts to promote HMOs are encouraging. Such efforts are based on data which recognize the potential of HMOs to alter patterns of use, particularly by replacing inpatient services with ambulatory care services and thereby reducing the overall cost of care.

Whether the prepaid group practice approach of HMOs permits more rational planning for use of health services (and therefore the possibility of a lower bed-to-population ratio), or whether the tighter limitation on bed supply forces hospitalization rates down, the result is the same. As Harris (1975) points out in his study on the effect of bed supply on hospital utilization:

> The results of this study support the contention that hospital beds tend to create their own demand for utilization, at least for the New York State counties studied. While this elaboration analysis was based only on New York State data, additional evidence from other areas are consistent with its results. It is generally recognized, for example, that pre-paid health insurance plans, such as those of Kaiser-Permanente in Oregon and California, maintain fewer beds per 1,000 of their subscribers than is the case for more conventionally insured populations, and that these plans have lower hospital utilization rates than more conventional plans (p. 171).

Physician Extenders. Similar efforts are underway to promote the use of physician extenders through experimental programs. The same amendments to the Social Security Act which provide the mechanism for incentive and prospective reimbursement experiments under Medicare as a way of encouraging hospital cost control also provide the mechanism for programs using physician extenders. The intent is to promote the use of lower-paid personnel who can substitute for direct physician services and thereby free the physicians for more complicated tasks.

Problems in the use of such extenders and associates include state-to-state differences in requirements for licensure and the permissible functions for such persons; malpractice insurance complications such as whether the physician superviser or the extender bears the responsibility; and general acceptance by both physicians and patients of such staff.

All of these various possible approaches relate to the need to deal with the overlapping problem areas of manpower provision, cost-financing, and availability of facilities and services at appropriate levels of care. Sound planning is obviously required to provide the coordination needed among providers to deal effectively with these problem areas. How successful has our planning been to date?

Klarman (1976) made the following observations:

> The primary reason for health planning in this country is the numerous instances in which the interests of the individual, health-care institution and those of the community may diverge, as in the case of hospital staff appointments for physicians.

> From a technical standpoint, it is much more difficult to plan for health services at the local level than nationally. Notwithstanding, health services are mostly provided at the local level, and health planning should be geared to the solution of local problems. In performing health planning, the local area can benefit from outside assistance.

> In the past decade, local health planning has been hampered by unstable federal funding. The absence of national policies and guidelines has led to a constant quest for new ideas. In the absence of substantive concerns, requirements for consumer representation have led to a preoccupation with structure and organization.

> What is required, in addition to steadier funding, is a fostering of local capabilities for health planning. Health planning organizations will require a good deal of technical assistance in the form of concrete ideas on ways to enhance the flexibility and versatility of health

facilities and personnel, monitoring natural experiments and learning their lessons, and elucidating the public policy implications of empirical research findings and even of apposite propositions from theory.

In specified circumstances the federal government is expected to serve as the superseding decision maker (p. 1).

OUTLOOK FOR THE FUTURE

In view of the data presented on projected demographic change, patterns and trends of use of health-related services and facilities, and the impact of various programs and developments on use, what changes can be anticipated for the delivery of health care services for the elderly?

The Short-Term Future. We anticipate that by 1985 the U.S. Congress will pass a national health insurance program. The program will not fully pay for the use of health services, in that there will be provisions for deductibles, coinsurance, and specified service exclusions, and there will be no greater exercise of control over the system for delivery of health care services. However there will be an improved standard of health insurance coverage for the entire population. With an improved guarantee of payment, the general population will place some greater demand on the health resources of this country, with a possible resultant downward pressure on the availability of health services for the aged. I do not anticipate that the alterations in overall demand caused by this insurance program will seriously erode the availability and use of health services by the elderly, but to the extent that there is an effect, it will be a negative one for the aged population. Existing coverage under private health insurance policies and public medical assistance programs will lessen the impact national health insurance might have had on the level of demand for health services from the population at large.

Over the next 10 years, health maintenance organizations will become increasingly popular and will serve as a mechanism for providing coordinated, comprehensive care not only for the aged but for all age groups. Fully packaged prepaid group plans which own and operate their own hospitals, extended care facilities, etc., should establish their potential value as devices to contain cost and hold down utilization, particularly of the more expensive inpatient facilities.

Physician extenders, physicians' assistants and associates, nurse practitioners, and whatever new titles may surface to designate these alter egos and limited replacements for physicians should come into greater use as a means of spreading the supply of physician services over a larger population base by the use of lower-paid, less highly trained personnel to deal with situations not requiring the physician's level of knowledge and skill.

Pressures from the government and other third-party payors for cost control and accountability in medical institutions should result in some improvement in the use of hospital care both in terms of average length of stay and rates of hospitalization. Since reduced rates of hospitalization often result in longer average lengths of stay, improvements in both dimensions will have to be monitored closely and dealt with as interrelated but separate entities. Concerns for cost control and appropriate use of the hospital as the most expensive facility should promote better use of a variety of care levels, including extended care facilities, outpatient ambulatory and day bed care services, and home health care. These would be used as a means to shorten or avoid hospital stays.

These various organizational and financial mechanisms are already in use or on the horizon. Between now and 1985, their use and acceptance should be expanded beyond the very limited scope which currently characterizes some of them. The next decade will probably not be one in which new ideas for the organization and delivery of medical care to the general population or to the aged are expounded. It will be a period of heightened awareness of our need to utilize more effectively our medical resources and manpower and to control the cost of medical care by putting into practice the various ideas on delivery system organization and financing which have been discussed over the last few decades. We have no dearth of ideas in this area. What we suffer from are limitations in our authority to direct the implementation of various delivery approaches, and limitations in our knowledge about which combinations will most effectively accomplish our dual purposes.

Efforts to promote experimentation with alternate implementation approaches and to provide the controls are already in evidence. The past decade has seen a variety of mechanisms for more rational planning of the provision and coordination of health services. We have seen such programs as Regional Medical Programs, Comprehensive Health Planning Agencies, Professional Standards Review Organizations, and a program of incentive and prospective reimbursement experiments under Medicare and Medicaid. The existence of such efforts to provide high quality medical care without waste of resources and intolerably high costs illustrates the degree of concern in these areas. During the next 10 years such efforts will be more successfully applied.

The picture presented for changes in the general structure of the health care delivery system over the next 10 years is one of movement along already defined lines. Health care for the aged will be more affected by these general developments than by changes in the age structure of the population. The adaptations needed in the health care delivery system to adjust to projected demographic changes should not require any drastic or concerted efforts. The changes will take place gradually and in total will comprise less of a change than was experienced over the past 25 years. The total number and proportion of the aged in society will be much larger and we cannot discount the impact of this change. However, accommodation to this increase should be manageable within a framework of normal changes in a market responding to altered need and demand patterns. These population changes will occur at a reasonable rate, and there is enough lead time to obviate the need for crash building or training programs. The direction and degree of change in general characteristics of the delivery system will be the most significant factor affecting the patterns of availability and use of health-related services and facilities for the aged.

The Next 25 Years. Much of the same pattern of development and interaction of factors can be predicted for the delivery of health-related services for the elderly between 1985 and 2000. The relative importance of changes in population and in organizational and financial arrangements on health care should be as described for the short-range future. The rate of change in population aged 65 and over will not be any different during the latter portion of this period. It will not be until past the year 2000 that the rate of population change and the overall distribution will be substantially altered.

The system for delivery of health-related services will not remain static during this period. The developmental patterns discussed above will mature and become institutionalized. However the realities of the political process and the accustomed practices and interests of providers and users will require accommodations over a period of time. These will be factors in the amount of time it takes for the expected changes to occur.

The system will probably remain pluralistic in terms of forms of delivery of health services. However there will be an increasing amount of care on a prepaid basis as opposed to fee-for-service, as well as increased reliance on physician extenders, etc. As a result of pressures for delivery of coordinated comprehensive care, and because of the problems of malpractice suits and insurance costs, physician-to-physician referral networks and self-policing of medical care practices will probably increase, as will the organizationally based practice of medicine. Efforts to contain costs and to rationalize the delivery of health care will result in increasing use of mechanisms for planning, coordination, and standards review, and methods of reimbursement which provide incentives for cost control. This can be done through local and regional planning and review groups and by applying positive and negative incentives to encourage certain measures and practices, or through more direct control over the medical care delivery system by the government.

It is in regard to the choice between these alternatives that I would like to propose a specific direction that should be taken in the delivery of health-related services. This direction would relate to the health care system in general, not to the aged in particular. However, as indicated, general attributes of the health care system will be more significant than anything else in the form taken by health services for the elderly. *A Proposal for Improving the Health Care Delivery System.* By the year 2000 the organizational trends discussed should be well established and no longer moving timidly into a realm of the private practice of medicine. Recognition of the need for planning, review, and coordination is currently well behind us, and in 25 years these functions will be increasingly accepted as necessary for the efficient and effective delivery of goods and services in an "industry" which will constitute, by then, at least 10 percent of our gross national product. The legitimacy of what are now tentative and basically cautious moves to put the medical care delivery system under greater control will be much more strongly affirmed. These moves may still be fought in some circles, but they will be acknowledged and justified openly as necessary to control an industry that is seriously in need of control.

It seems apparent, however, that providing the stimulus and structure for self-control is not enough to produce the rational system of care delivery needed to serve the best interests of the general population. These mechanisms have been effectively co-opted by elements of the industry to serve their own interests and needs. This development is not surprising, given the planning partnerships that have been established and the lack of specific guidelines for evaluating performance and results.

What is the missing ingredient in such efforts? There is no real measure of direct public control over the delivery system for medical care. By the year 2000, there will have to be direct public control, in at least a limited sphere of activity, over the medical care delivery system in this country. At a minimum, this control will have to operate on two levels.

Responsibility for overall policy should be centralized. It would include planning for resource development, manpower training, resource allocation between regional or local areas, and establishment of guidelines for coordination and use of the various major levels of health care. This should facilitate the implementation of new knowledge gained through studies in the areas of incentives to cost control, optional organizational arrangements, interrelationships among facilities and levels of care (whether parts of HMOs or as separate entities), and the use of various medical care personnel such as physician extenders and nurse practitioners.

Responsibilities for coordinating the various providers of medical care should be placed at the regional or local level, since direct delivery of care is performed at the local level. This coordination should be exercised to control the unwarranted duplication and overlap of services and facilities among units at the same and different levels of care, as well as to control the inappropriate use of various levels of care. The availability of and access to needed care modalities can also be most effectively handled at the regional or local levels.

The implementation of such controls can probably most reasonably be accomplished by incorporating them within the structure of the national health insurance program which should be in place and have a base of operating experience well before the year 2000. I do not think that authorization for a national health insurance program with any meaningful level of direct control can be passed as an initial piece of legislation. These controls will be added later as experience under the program reaffirms the data from the Medicare experience that a system to guarantee payment which exercises no direct control over the delivery system cannot accomplish its purposes with or without cost containment.

What are the explicit and implicit purposes of such a program? Explicitly, it is intended to remove the financial barriers to health care through the insurance mechanism of guaranteed payment for care received; implicitly, it is intended to stimulate the availability of care appropriate to the health needs of the population.

It is in stimulating the availability of appropriate care that direct system control should have its major impact on the delivery of health-related care for the elderly. The provision of coordinated, comprehensive care is of greatest concern in the area of chronic disease. Although the aged share the need for all forms of health care, it is in the need for long-term care for the chronic diseases that they are most vulnerable. This aspect of care will benefit most from direct system control overseeing the availability of, and access to, needed forms of care which are appropriately coordinated.

Health care for the elderly will also be affected by the general dimensions of the changes envisioned and the program developments recommended here. Current patterns of utilization and pressures on existing facilities may be altered dramatically because of better coordination among providers of care and more appropriate use of the various levels of care. This may be possible without any alteration at the individual level in the overall need for care or in quality of care standards.

The form health care for the elderly takes by the year 2000 will be more subject to changes within the system for delivering and financing health care in general than to any specific steps taken to deal with the growth of the aged population or to satisfy their health care needs as a single segment of our society.

REFERENCES

Andersen, R. & Anderson, O. W. *A decade of health services: Social survey trends in use and expenditures.* Chicago: University of Chicago Press, 1967.

Coe, R. M. & Brehm, H. P. *Preventive health care for adults.* New Haven: College and University Press Services, 1972.

Coe, R. M., Brehm, H. P. & Peterson, W. H. Impact of Medicare on the organization of community health resources. *The Milbank Memorial Fund Quarterly*, 1974, *52*(3), 231–264.

Davis, K. Equal treatment and unequal benefits: The Medicare program. *The Milbank Memorial Fund Quarterly*, 1975, *53*(4), 449–488.

Harris, D. M. An elaboration of the relationship between general hospital bed supply and general hospital utilization. *Journal of Health and Social Behavior*, 1975, *16*(2), 163–172.

Klarman, H. E. National policies and local planning for health services. *The Milbank Memorial Fund Quarterly*, 1976, *54*(1), 1–28.

National Center for Health Statistics. *Characteristics of residents in institutions for the aged and chronically ill, U.S.—April–June 1963*, Series 12, No. 2. Washington, D.C.: National Center for Health Statistics, 1965.

National Center for Health Statistics. *Characteristics of residents in nursing and personal care homes, U.S.—June–August 1969*, Series 12, No. 19. Washington, D.C.: National Center for Health Statistics, 1973.

National Center for Health Statistics. *Physician visits,* Series 10, No. 97. Washington, D.C.: National Center for Health Statistics, 1975.

U.S. Department of Commerce, Bureau of the Census. *Pocket data book, USA 1969,* Washington, D.C.: U.S. Government Printing Office, 1969.

U.S. Department of Commerce, Bureau of the Census. *Population estimates and projections,* Series P 25, No. 601. October 1975.

U.S. Department of Commerce, Bureau of the Census. *Statistical abstract of the U.S. 1970* (91st annual edition). Washington, D.C.: U.S. Government Printing Office, 1970.

U.S. Department of Health, Education and Welfare, *Compendium of national health expenditure data.* DHEW Pub. No. (SSA76–11927). Washington, D.C.: U.S. Department of Health, Education and Welfare, 1976a.

U.S. Department of Health, Education and Welfare, *Medicare, Fiscal Years 1969–1973.* Selected state data. DHEW Pub. No. (SSA76–11711), Washington, D.C.: Social Security Administration, 1976b.

West, H. Five years of Medicare—A statistical review. *Social Security Bulletin,* 1971, *34*(12), 17–27.

-8-

The Future of Health-Related Care for the Elderly in Europe

Esther Ammundsen

Generalizations about European health care are not easily formulated. The great diversity of politics, economics, traditions, health, and social systems among the European nations makes it difficult to predict how the Continent as a whole will provide health-related care for the elderly in the future. The effort is further complicated because the problems facing the older generation are rarely health problems alone or socioeconomic problems alone, but most often a combination of the two. Nonetheless, the effort is worthwhile because it may offer insight both to countries outside Europe and to individual European nations.

Age Structures in European Countries. The process must begin with an examination of the demographic picture and what changes are projected. Determining the number of people currently in the older age groups and how many are expected to join those ranks in the future is, of course, a prerequisite to determining the amount of health-related care which should be made available.

At the present time the age structures of the various European regions differ substantially. Northern and Western Europe are much "older" than other European regions, as Figures 1 and 2 indicate. The Soviet Union is currently the "youngest." By the year 2000, however, these differences will be nearly eliminated. The figures also show that the 60 and over age group will diminish through the remainder of the 1970s and the beginning of the 1980s, especially in Eastern and Central Europe (excluding the Soviet Union). However a similar decrease is not projected for the over-75 group, so that the relative number of the very old will continue to increase for some years. The person who attains age 65 can currently expect to live another fifteen years.

It is evident that Europe will continue to grapple with the problems of providing adequate health-related care for a sub-

Figure 1   Percentage of the Total European Population Over 60 (*Recent demographic trends in Europe and the outlook until the year 2000.* 1974).

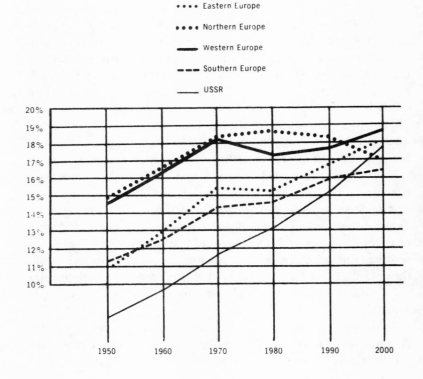

Figure 2 **Percentage of the Total European Population Over 75** (*Recent demographic trends in Europe and the outlook until the year 2000. 1974*).

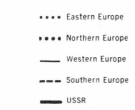

• • • • Eastern Europe

▸ • • • Northern Europe

——— Western Europe

— — — Southern Europe

▬▬▬ USSR

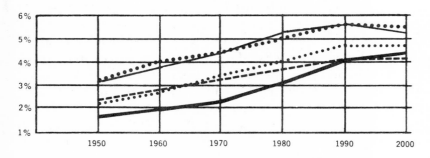

stantial number of older people. Many factors contribute to making provision of such care a difficult problem: early retirement, greater demand on public services, urbanization, labor market variability, and shortages of housing. For example, recent widespread unemployment in many European countries has seriously hampered all the well-intended efforts to ease the abrupt change from active working life to retirement by providing part-time employment for older people. The picture is further complicated by the tendency toward longer periods of education, which is reducing the number of active working years.

The Financing of Health and Health-Related Care. The serious economic picture of recent years has had an overwhelming influence upon the extent and type of health-related care currently available or planned for the future. In contrast to the booming 60s, when appropriations for innumerable social programs and services were readily available, particularly in Denmark, the 70s have offered only lean budgets and cutbacks on the expenses incurred through the optimistic management prevailing a decade ago.

Answers to the question "How is the care of the older generation financed in Europe?" are kaleidoscopic in their variations. There are a number of studies on the financing of such care, but an overall picture or description is lacking and will be very difficult to procure.

The World Health Organization's Regional Office for Europe is contemplating the development of a description of service policies in Europe. However the difficulties of such a task are enormous. Many authorities and organizations in each country are involved in this field; as a consequence, little or no central statistical knowledge exists, and the constantly changing conditions and approaches of each European country make a thorough assessment of service policies almost immediately outdated. The Commission of European Communities has undertaken the task of describing social service policies in the Common Market countries, but it has yet to publish its findings.

The issue of private versus public financing for elderly health care has been an important one. During the latter half of this century, the traditional responsibility for the older family members in many countries has—to varying degrees—shifted from family and private assistance to the public sector. Although domestic family assistance is still provided in all European countries, the farther one goes north and east, the more it is taken over by public authorities and financed by taxes.

Administrative Patterns. The administrative pattern of elderly health care can vary from an almost complete centralization of service planning and delivery functions (which is very rare), to a complete decentralization of authority with the entire responsibility (including financial responsibility in some cases) resting with local authorities.

INTEGRATION OF HEALTH AND SOCIAL SERVICES. The varying relations between health services and social services also cause complications. There is no common practice distinguishing which services belong to the health service realm with its hospitals, nurses, physicians, and therapists, and which services come under the authority of the social services and their old age pensions, additional subsidies, assistance by social workers, meals on wheels, sheltered housing, and old-age homes. One also finds all patterns of services, from complete integration to complete separation. In some countries integration exists at the central level and separation at the local level; in others the converse is true. This diversity of operations makes exchange of meaningful information between nations very difficult. Even two countries as similar as Sweden and Denmark have difficulties. For example, in Sweden the hospital authorities are partly responsible for the long-term care institutions (annex hospitals), whereas in Denmark the responsibility for the chronically ill and disabled rests with the social authorities (nursing homes).

The reasons for these differences are mainly historical and traditional. However, once established, practices become extremely difficult to change, even if everyone sees and admits the desirability of a better integration. Nevertheless, in many European countries the social and health authorities have become better coordinated during the last 10 to 15 years. Simultaneously, the tendency toward public financing of services has grown.

COMPONENTS OF CARE. The systems of health-related care which have been built up during the latter part of this century fall into three categories:

1. Institutional care, consisting of special hospital beds for the aged (located in geriatric and long-term care departments or special hospitals), institutions (nursing homes) especially intended as permanent residences for the disabled and sick, and old people's homes intended for persons who do not require nursing assistance. All three kinds of institutions are inpatient facilities, but there are varying patterns and standards among the different European countries.

2. Publicly financed home care consisting of home nurses, home helpers, home visitors, and several specialized groups such as occupational therapists and physiotherapists, chiropodists, and others who, to an increasing extent, replace domestic family care. Home care is supplemented to varying degrees with economic and social benefits. For

example, in addition to a pension, the government may provide subsidies for housing, transportation, meals, etc., which are only indirectly health-related.

3. Sheltered housing of several different types, often in modern apartment buildings, where services such as cleaning, food preparation, supervision, and perhaps some form of temporary nursing care are available. The rent for this type of housing is often subsidized. In this area the United States' progress surpasses that of other countries in the old world.

The different forms of public health-related care have been briefly described above. However, in most European countries, public care is mixed with a more or less widespread private system. The private system includes completely independent and self-financed institutions, as well as privately planned and operated institutions with total public reimbursement of expenses (but often without public influence).

NEGLECT OF PRIMARY CARE. In too many countries the role of general practitioners has been reduced in recent years. Where available, they are the normal and primary health contact for all age groups including those over 65. Primary health care has the greatest significance for the health of this older population group but is often overlooked because "elderly care" is thought of solely as services especially designed for the elderly or related to the old-age pension. For older people, the failure of so many countries to maintain a good system of primary health care and to provide for adequate numbers of general practitioners is no less than a catastrophe.

TRENDS FOR THE FUTURE

The following appear to be future European trends in the field of health-related care for the elderly:

1. An increased proportion of services for the elderly will be financed through public means or perhaps compulsory state-subsidized insurance systems.

2. The pressing economic situation will make any expansion of service systems difficult. This particularly applies to institutional care, which is by far the most expensive of all services.

3. Interest in studying ways and means to replace institutional care by home care or sheltered housing will continue to grow. Suggestions that families be paid to provide care for their own older members indicate the seriousness of public concern over institutionalization.

4. Measures to activate the older generation and to delay the development of disability and dependency by identifying high-risk groups and treating them in time to prevent diseases and impairments are constantly discussed but have made only a modest start.

5. Present systems for providing the necessary fare for those who need it have been determined more by accidental factors than by careful planning: since the family could not or would not take care of its older members, something else had to be done. Voluntary organizations set up either by religious orders, trade associations, or other bodies were already in existence and wanted to (and could) do at least part of the work. Pressure groups grew up among the professions working with the health care problems and seeing the need for action. In many places it became politically popular to "do something for the older generation" and to win some votes in the process.

All these factors tended to make services grow in a rather haphazard way. However during recent years the problem of providing such services has grown too large to approach casually. The services are also becoming too expensive, even if the total costs are masked because of the complicated method of apportioning financing among state government, local government, and private sources. In many places recipients find the resulting service programs unsatisfactory. In other areas the question of whether the services rendered really meet the needs (or the demands) of the elderly remains unanswered, and unfortunately, in practically all localities, older persons' involvement in and influence upon the planning and delivery of the services seems to be minimal.

Need for Epidemiological Research. The essential question is—What do we really know about the population group for whom these special services have been or are being planned? Although there are enormous amounts of literature (gerontological, geriatric, general medical, public health, social and sociological), we are still very short of the kind of epidemiological research that could shed some light on some of the questions presently facing public health and social administrators:

1. How many of the elderly really need special age-related services and how many can be served satisfactorily by the regular health services?

2. At what age does the greater demand for special care appear?

3. How many still need the most expensive care (institutional), and how can these people be located?

4. What is the present utilization of existing health and social services in this age group?

5. Can anything more be done to identify special risk groups, diseases, and conditions which could be treated before it is too late and thus postpone disability and physical or mental dependency?

In recent years several European institutes and centers have begun to address these problems, but so far very little of this research has been published. Because this field is so subject to rapid political, economic, and administrative changes, it seems best to concentrate in this chapter on a few very recent studies.

Insights Provided by Recent Research in Sweden and Scotland. One essential factor in estimating the demand for health-related services is public opinion and attitudes. In general, many European countries have painted the picture of aging much too bleakly. Very often the older generation is viewed as a homogeneous group with health needs different from those of people under 65 but with roughly the same needs and demands throughout the 65-plus group. It is also commonly believed that a very large proportion of the elderly population is in institutions or ought to be. The elderly are seen as lonely, depressed people complaining of bodily pain and feeling cut off from society, as they are often cut off from work. The psychological impact of these attitudes should not be underestimated. Everyone has a tendency to comply with the role expected of him, and if society expects the elderly to fulfill the narrow, negative role described above, older people will ask themselves, "Why try to be active and optimistic?"

Sociological and medical research has indicated that the current situation for the older population is not as bad as the public believes, but only recently, and in limited areas, do the research findings seem to be penetrating public opinion.

A more accurate portrayal of the European elderly is offered by the recent research of Svanborg et al. (1975), who are working on an epidemiological population-based description of the somatic, mental, and social status of 70-year-olds in Gothenburg, Sweden, and by the work of Gruer (1975), who has made a population-based, age-divided study of older persons living in a semirural district in Scotland.

Gruer's Scottish study (Figures 3 and 4) shows that the number of medical conditions increases with advanced age, especially after age 75. Although the findings in Svanborg's Swedish study have not yet been completely published, preliminary reports present a picture somewhat like the Scottish 70 to 74 age group.

Both these and earlier studies seem to show that the older persons are inclined to underestimate or accept their symptoms, so that relative optimism and contentment are much more common than generally believed (Figure 5). In addition, both studies found that loneliness, which the public believes to be a common state among the elderly, is actually relatively uncommon (Figures 5 and 6).

Such research may provide some answers to the problem of identifying risk groups and introducing preventive measures. The follow-up to the Swedish study (which began in 1976 when treatment and measures were instituted where indicated) will be most interesting.

Figure 3   Age and Number of Medical Conditions Recorded in the Scottish Sample (Gruer, 1975).

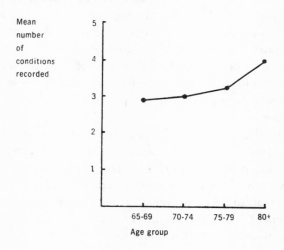

Utilization of Health-Related Services in Three Countries.
Bearing in mind the great diversity of European health care systems, an examination of the present utilization of health-related services in Denmark, Scotland, and Sweden should be helpful in assessing the future need for such services. Present utilization may be categorized in three ways: (1) institutional care (long-term hospitals, nursing homes, and old-age homes); (2) general practitioners or other primary medical services; and (3) home nurses, home helpers, etc. Table 8.1 shows some relevant Danish institutional figures.

In Denmark the so-called nursing homes—the backbone of the institutional care—do not rely on any payments by the home residents or charity. In other words, none are totally private homes. All institutions are fully subsidized, operated, and controlled by public authorities. If an elderly person in need of institutional care has private means of financing his care, the person is allowed to keep his or her capital intact, but must pay up to 60 percent of his or her interest and other income. However, this is the case for less than 10 percent of all nursing home residents.

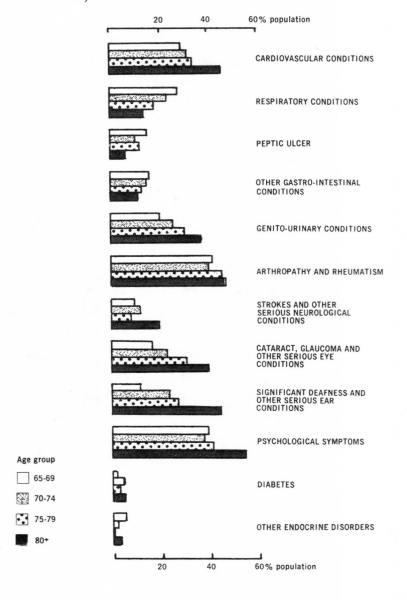

Figure 5 Age and Outlook in the Scottish Sample (Gruer, 1975).

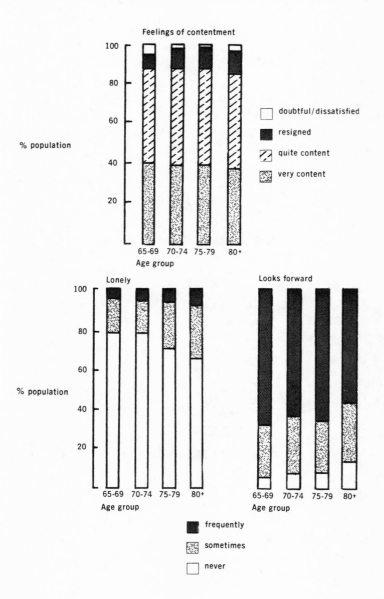

Figure 6   Outlook for 70-year-olds in the Swedish Sample (Svanborg, 1975).

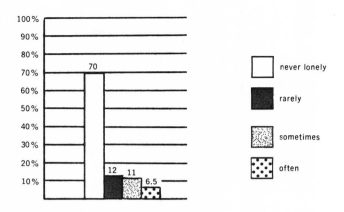

Figures 7 and 8 show the total number and percentages of those institutionalized in Denmark during 1965–1968 and 1975 (respectively, 5.8 percent and 6.8 percent of the population over 65 years of age). The diagrams show clearly that under the age of 75, only a small percentage of the population concerned lives in these institutions (in the age group 70–74, only 2.41 percent). Within the general hospital system ("acute hospitals") some 1,200 to 1,500 persons are now awaiting transfer to nursing homes, compared to a total of about 44,000 already living in these institutions. The corresponding Swedish figure for the number of 70-year-olds institutionalized in Gothenburg is 3 percent (Table 8.2).

ROLE OF PRIMARY CARE.   In regard to the use of primary health care personnel, the Scottish study concludes that the general practitioner is the individual best able both to know the older person's needs and to deliver the necessary care. The Swedish study reached a similar finding. The high levels of such contact in Scotland (Table 8.3) and Sweden (Table 8.4) indicate that the role of the general practitioner (or other primary medical service) has been grossly underestimated.

Table 8.1 Elderly Population and Nursing Home Beds in Denmark

	1962	1968	1975
Total population (millions)	4.647	4.867	5.054
Percentage of population 65 and over	10.9	11.9	13.3
Number of beds in nursing- and old-age homes (occupancy: circa 95%)	28,500	32,500	46,800
Beds per 1000 inhabitants over 65	-	58	70
Personnel per bed	-	about 0.4	0.7

Figure 7   Total Number of Residents in Nursing and Old-Age Homes in Denmark (Olson, 1975).

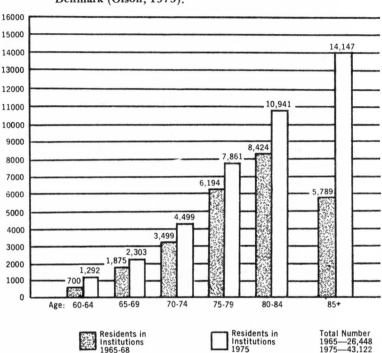

ROLE OF HOME HEALTH SERVICES.   A quantitative estimate of the different types of home-help services is very difficult, if not impossible, to make. Such services often replace the private assistance previously extended by family, neighbors, and friends. A recent estimate by the municipality of Copenhagen (Dalgaard, 1977), where home helpers have existed for many years, is that approximately 24 percent of the population over 65 will need these services in the coming years. The Swedish study found that a slightly smaller proportion—18 percent—currently required assistance with home care (Table 8.2).

Even in Denmark, where practically all expenses are paid by public funds from state, counties, and municipalities, the total cost of these elderly health-related services is difficult to estimate;

Figure 8   Percentage of the Population in Nursing and Old-Age Homes
            in Denmark (Olson, 1975).

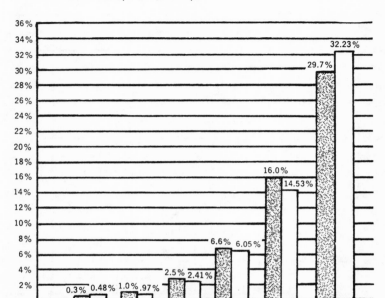

in countries where private sources contribute to elderly care, a
cost assessment is nearly impossible (Harlem, 1974).

ROLE OF INSTITUTIONAL CARE.   The cost of the most expensive form of elderly care, institutional care, is more readily identi-
fiable. Currently, a bed in a Danish nursing home costs from
$20,000 to $25,000 per year to maintain. How many institutional
beds are really needed? This is a difficult question to answer,
depending as it does on preference and upon availability of both
institutional and home-based services. During the last 25 years,
estimates of need in Denmark have ranged from 1.5 to 24 percent
of the population over 65. Presently, institutional beds are available for approximately 7 percent of the 65-plus population. This
latter figure is probably realistic, provided that (1) the geograph-

Table 8.2 Characteristics of 70-Year-Old Persons in Sweden

	%
Institutionalized in a medical or social ward	3
Live in their homes	97
Need daily assistance with personal care, dressing, etc.	2
Need assistance with home care	18
Receive public home service (of all who need assistance)	50
Receive private assistance (of all who need assistance)	30
Receive assistance from children (of all who need assistance)	9

Source: Svanborg (1975).

Table 8.3 Contacts of Scottish Elderly Persons with General Practitioner (GP), Health Visitor (HV), and District Nurse (DN)[a]

Time of last contact	Percentage having contact with		
	G.P	H.V	D.N.
1 week	11.5	0.4	4.7
1 week – 1 month	19.4	0.1	1.1
1 month– 3 months	20.6	0.3	1.1
3 months +	47.3	0.3	1.9
Unknown	1.2	0.1	0.3
No contact	–	98.8	91.0
	100.0	100.0	100.1

[a]Total number excluding those in long-stay hospitals = 742.
Source: Gruer (1975).

Table 8.4   Contacts of Swedish Elderly Persons with Physician or Ambulatory Hospital

	%
4 times or more per year	24
1-3 times per year	35
Less than 1 time per year	26
Never	15
	100

Source: Svanborg (1975).

ical distribution corresponds to local needs; (2) only those who really need nursing home care are taken into the institutions (against which rule many sins are committed); (3) there is supplementary provision for some psychiatric cases, and (4) external social and medical assistance is sufficient.

If these provisions are not fulfilled, the reliance on institutional care (which may often be the easiest, although not the best solution for the individual) will automatically increase.

Conclusion.   In Denmark, as in other Scandinavian countries, the health-care system and its problems have gone through the development which many European countries either have seen or will experience. Initially there were no provisions for care except in the case of real destitution; then there was a period in which health-related care was financed and influenced by private sources; and finally there has been a period of growing and eventual total public responsibility for health care services. During a period of strong propaganda about the establishment of better and more elaborate institutions, the public has become convinced that practically all older people will eventually need this type of care.

What is needed at this juncture is a good assessment of current alternatives and a thorough calculation of total costs of institutional care, as well as of other forms of care. In the future, replacement of some of the existing institutional care with better developed home care and sheltered housing will undoubtedly be in the interest of both the elderly and the ministers of finance.

As noted earlier, the World Health Organization's Regional Office for Europe, headquartered in Copenhagen, is planning to develop a knowledge-gathering program—knowledge which will enable WHO to advise governments fully and accurately on the planning and organizing of elderly health-related services (World Health Organization, 1974).

The first steps in such a program would be (1) the multinational launching of epidemiological research similar to the studies mentioned earlier (although possibly less extensive); and (2) the development of a description of existing service patterns for the European elderly. It is hoped that these two activities will help accelerate the service planning processes in both developed and developing countries.

The close coordination of planning, implementation, and research within the field of health-related care for the elderly, which touches so many aspects of human life, is an absolute imperative. Medical doctors alone, or economists alone, or social scientists alone, cannot possibly provide an accurate picture for the decision makers who will have the final say about the conditions under which this generation and coming generations will spend a considerable part of their lives.

REFERENCES

Dalgaard, O.Z. Growth of services for care and assistance for old people in the municipality of Copenhagen from 1967 to the energy crisis in 1974. *Ugeskrift for Laeger,* 1977, *139,* 491–503.

Gruer, R. Needs of the elderly in the Scottish borders. Scottish Health Service Studies, 1975, *33.*

Harlem, G. *The health protection of the elderly.* Regional Committee for Europe, WHO, EUR/RC24/Techn. Disc./1. Bucharest, 1974.

Olsen, H. Old people living in nursing and old-age homes. Copenhagen: Danish National Institute of Social Research, 1975, *57*.

Recent demographic trends in Europe and the outlook until the year 2000. Brussels: Secretariat of the Economic Commission for Europe, 1974.

Svanborg, A., et al. Seventy-year-old people in Gothenburg. A population study in an industrialized Swedish city. Published in part. *Acta Medica Scandinavica,* 1975, *198*.

World Health Organization. Planning and organization of geriatric services. Report of a WHO Expert Committee. Techn. Rep. Ser. 548, WHO. Geneva: 1974.

-9-

Trends in the Development of Services for the Aging Under the Older Americans Act

Robert C. Benedict

The Older Americans Act of 1965 is in many respects representative of other categorical social welfare legislation produced by the predominantly Democratic Congress following the watershed years of the Roosevelt Administration. The act expresses the hopes and the aspirations of a population traditionally at the fringe of American life. Since its enactment, it has addressed a variety of service problems incrementally, as consumer organizations, social service agencies, bureaucrats, and legislators sought changes reflecting their particular needs and interests. Only rarely has there been sufficient consensus to force significant changes either in the scope of programs administered under the act, or in the scale of resources authorized by the Congress to implement its provisions.

The Older Americans Act contains a host of dichotomies characteristic of other social legislation. Philosophically, the act is an expression of the belief that governmental intervention can enhance the well-being of a whole class of people. Conversely, it contains subtle exclusions which reflect an uncertain commitment and an unwillingness or an inability to address fundamental questions of authority and resources. The legislation is a prime example of the modern juxtaposition of rising expectations for governmental solutions and fear of excessive governmental involvement in our daily lives.

This chapter examines the emerging trends and developments of services for the aging under the Older Americans Act of 1965, focusing on the future of the act as an instrument of national social policy. Projecting the future of the Older Americans Act over the next 10 to 25 years requires that we focus briefly on those social conditions and circumstances which have generated support for the act. An attempt is made to trace the evolution of its major provisions in order to determine the extent to which it has achieved its aims. The chapter concludes with speculations about the future of social programs for the elderly.

To develop an empirical base from which to evaluate observations on the short-range and long-range future of programs for older people under the act, a group of experts was invited to speculate on this legislation's future directions. In March 1976, 25 persons were invited to respond to the following questions:

1. With respect to the Older Americans Act of 1965, what did we expect and what did we get?
2. In the short run, can tinkering help? What changes should be made over the next 5 to 10 years?
3. In the long run, (25–50 years), does the act have a future? Is it or can it be important to older people?
4. Of the changing political, economic, social, and demographic forces, which stand out in your mind as the most critical factors to be considered in reshaping social programs for the aging?

The respondents included current and former federal officials who have been charged with the implementation of the Older Americans Act, members of the academic community who have been closely associated with the act, and representatives of national organizations who have formed the basis of political support for the act.

The respondents included Elias Cohen, University of Pennsylvania; Nelson Cruikshank, National Council of Senior Citizens;

Wilma Donahue, International Center for Social Gerontology; Carroll Estes, University of California at San Francisco; Byron Gold, University of Chicago; Leonard Gottesman, Philadelphia Geriatric Center; Hobart Jackson, Stephen Smith Geriatric Center; Norman Lourie, Deputy Secretary for Federal Policy, Pennsylvania Department of Public Welfare; John Martin, American Association of Retired Persons and former U.S. Commissioner on Aging; Jack Ossofsky, National Council on the Aging; and Herbert Shore, Executive Vice-President, Golden Acres Nursing Home, Dallas, Texas.

Antecedents to the New Law.   The primary factors which led to the passage of the Older Americans Act of 1965 were the poverty and disability that marked the lives of an expanding population of older people. Since the passage of Title I of the Social Security Act of 1935, income maintenance caseworkers had been confronted with the myriad of social problems of the elderly poor. Our long-standing reliance on income maintenance and related casework services, county homes, alms-houses, mental hospitals, and boarding homes was found to be unjustified in the era of rising expectations which followed World War II. Social scientists continued to document widespread poverty, disability, and dependence among the elderly in spite of general improvements in the standard of living among American families as a whole.

DISABILITY AND DEPENDENCY DATA.   According to vital and health statistics compiled by the United States Public Health Services (National Center for Health Statistics, 1971), 86 percent of all elderly persons suffer from one or more chronic conditions. Although the large majority of elderly are not impeded in the conduct of major activities, some are. The incidence of serious disability increases significantly with age. Among the noninstitutionalized, fewer than 15 percent of those 45 to 64 report any limitation in major activities due to disease or impairment. At age 65 and over, nearly 40 percent report such limitation, and approximately 14 percent are totally unable to carry out major activities.

Relating specific instances of impairment to age group indicates a significant correlation between age and impairment among those 65 and over. At ages 65 to 69, 9 percent report serious difficulty "getting about the house." At 75 to 79 this figure rises to 15 percent, and at 85 plus to 34 percent of the noninstitutionalized elderly. At ages 65 to 69, 4 percent of the elderly report serious difficulty washing and bathing; by ages 75 to 79, 8 percent report difficulties, and for those 80 and over the proportion is 23 percent. Among those 65 to 69, 15 percent report that they are "hard of hearing"; among those 75 to 79, this was true of 25 percent. At 80-plus the rate soars to 54 percent of all noninstitutionalized elderly persons. At 65 to 69, 11 percent of the elderly report serious difficulty walking. The proportion gradually rises to 20 percent among those 75 to 79. At age 80-plus, 37 percent of the noninstitutionalized elderly report serious difficulty in walking.

Data of this kind began to appear in the 1950s, after the first National Conference on Aging. Its interpretation led to conclusions that provided the basis for our current national social policies. Experts concluded that the problems of the elderly, in some respects at least, are peculiar to the physiological, sociological, and psychological aspects of the aging process and cannot be ameliorated by income maintenance alone. They agreed that the problems are characteristic of an aging population and are not residual. Adjustments can be made in health services, social services, and living arrangements to improve the quality of living for older people, but basic problems will persist as long as the elderly constitute a significant population group. Finally, they concluded that the problems are of such magnitude that they require the significant commitment of substantial public resources at all levels of government.

Early Development and Support. The Kennedy-Johnson years represented an extraordinary period of hopefulness and optimism. A chronology of the social legislation of that era dramatically documents the national sense of high expectation. The Civil Rights Act of 1964, the establishment of the Peace Corps, the Economic Opportunity Act of 1964, the enactment of Medicare and Medicaid in 1965, the Food Stamp Act of 1964, the Urban Mass Transportation Act of 1964, the Vocational Education Act of 1963, the Community Mental Health legislation, the

development of special housing programs, and the 1967 amendments to the social services titles of the Social Security Act are
only a few examples of far-reaching legislation enacted during
that period. The Detroit riots were still in the future, the Vietnam
War was only a shadow on the national conscience, and scarcity
was only an academic principle. The economy had not begun its
long decline, and no one worried about fuel oil or gasoline shortages. A rising national recognition of the aging as a class of
people with unique problems coupled with the emergence of
national organizations as advocates for increased governmental
support provided the impetus for enactment of the Older Americans Act in 1965. A description of the act is provided below.

THE FIRST 10 YEARS (1965–1975)

In many respects, the Older Americans Act was a continuation of
a national planning and development exercise begun at the first
White House Conference on Aging in 1961. The Conference
report (1961) provided much of the data and recommendations
from which the legislation was drafted. The language of the report and the act reflects quite well the state of our knowledge and
experience at that time. Our goals were expressed in general
terms with a focus on planning processes at the federal, state, and
local levels. Although there were statements of the need for
specific social services, they could not be expressed quantita-
tively. Neither the White House Conference nor the act established any basis for major service programs. Both focused instead
on the development of planning processes in federal, state, and
local governments.

The perceptions of those responding to the think-tank exercise
about the first 10 years of experience under the Older Americans
Act clustered around four general themes:

1. The act was an historic symbol of a national policy commitment to meeting the social needs of older people.
2. This was a period of planning and organizational development at all levels of government.

3. This was also a period of experimentation and demonstration which brought definition to social services concepts in the field of aging.

4. The absence of adequate information, data, and knowledge in early phases greatly hampered efforts to evaluate performance and to provide directions for the future.

The Older Americans Act as a National Policy Statement. The respondents to the think-tank exercise had a variety of reactions to the significance of the Older Americans Act as a national policy statement. One respondent pointed out the symbolic importance of the passage of the act: "There was hope and, in some quarters, the belief that passage of an Older Americans Act would mean a new dawn for America's senior citizens." This respondent stressed the importance of the declaration of objectives set forth in Title I as the most significant title in the act. It may be of some use to restate the key passages of Title I.

The Congress hereby finds and declares that the older people of our Nation are *entitled to, and it is the joint duty and responsibility of the Governments of the United States and of the several States and their political subdivisions to assist our older people to secure equal opportunity to the full and free enjoyment of the following objectives:* (1) An adequate income in retirement . . . (2) the best possible physical and mental health . . . (3) suitable housing . . . (4) full restorative services . . . (5) pursuit of meaningful activity . . . (8) efficient community services, including access to low-cost transportation . . . (9) immediate benefit from proven research knowledge . . . (10) freedom, independence, and the free exercise of individual initiative in planning and managing their own lives. [Italics added]

This is an extraordinary declaration. What was the Congressional intent of this declaration? What level of government is to be held accountable for the well-being of older people? Does it constitute entitlement for each and every older American or mere Congressional boastfulness?

Respondents seemed to have two distinct reactions to the act. One group perceived its primary purpose as the establishment of pre-eminent policy-making organizations at the state and national level. This group saw a symbolic significance in the act, believing that it represented Congress's recognition of old peo-

Table 9.1 The Development of the Older Americans Act of 1965

Title	Description and Purpose as of 1976	Major Historical Trends and Changes
Title I	Declaration of Objective	*(1965)* A basic statement of social policy objectives for serving older people stated in quality of life terms such as adequate income, suitable housing, physical and mental health, employment opportunity, community services. *(1973)* Included "access to low cost transportation" and a new section focusing on "comprehensiveness," poverty, coordination, planning, and consumer participation.
Title II	Administration on Aging	*(1965)* Established the Administration on Aging in the Department of Health, Education and Welfare, creating the position of Commissioner appointed by the Secretary. *(1973)* Revised Title II placing AoA in the Office of the Secretary, making the Commissioner directly responsible to the Secretary, prohibiting the Secretary from otherwise delegating AoA powers, expanding the coordinating role of AoA in the federal government, and creating the Federal Council on Aging.
Title III	Grants for State and Community Programs on Aging	*(1965)* Original Title: Grants for Community Planning, Services and Training; formula grants to states for community services demonstrations, establishment of State Agencies on Aging, local project support limited to three years in diminishing proportions of 75% (1st), 60% (2nd) and 50% (3rd).

(1969) Permitted fourth and subsequent year funding by the states at 50%. Section 305 added establishing authority for Areawide Model Projects. Federal support for state administration increased to $75,000. *(1973)* Major amendments establishing authority for creating Planning and Service Areas in the states, and requiring the establishment of Area Agencies on Aging, and the preparation of Area Plans for the development and coordination of comprehensive services for aging. *(1974)* Section 309 added providing for special transportation services.

Title IV — Training and Research

(1965) Originally Title V, from 1965 to 1973 limited to training only. In 1973 the authority was expanded to include Research and Development (Part B) and the establishment of Multidisciplinary Centers of Gerontology (Part C).

Title V — Multipurpose Senior Centers

(1973) Added as Title V and providing for the acquisition, altering, or renovation of facilities to serve as multipurpose senior centers. Funds appropriated for the first time in 1976.

Title VI — National Older Americans Volunteer Program

(1969) The Retired Senior Volunteer Program and the Foster Grandparent Program were administered by the Administration on Aging until transferred to ACTION in 1971.

Title VII — Nutrition Program for the Elderly

(1973) Grants to states for the purpose of making grants to communities for nutrition and supportive services for persons aged 60 and over.

Title VIII	Rescinded	
Title IX	Community Services Employment	*(1973)* Enacted in 1973 as Title IX of the Older Americans Comprehensive Service Amendments. Not part of the Older Americans Act of 1965 as amended. Added to the Older Americans Act in 1975.

ple as a distinct population group with persistent social problems.

The other group viewed the act primarily as an impetus for the development of community-based social services for older people. Many of these respondents emphasized the importance of the 1973 amendments which formalized the development of community planning and service agencies.

Both these views are compatible with the proposition that the major impact of the act has been its formation of organizations. Our society has often achieved change through the influence of organization. Every public and privately conceived cause has given rise to complex and purposeful organizations. In this sense the Older Americans Act is very much in keeping with the development of education, health, and social programs in this century. The trend has been toward the slow but methodical establishment of an intrenched organizational infrastructure, organized as a loose confederation within the existing structure of our federal and state governments, around the common goal of well-being for older people. One respondent described the Administration on Aging as a locomotive set in motion in some largely unknown direction, with its staff laying track just ahead of the moving engine. The one fundamental accomplishment of the first 10 years may have been the spreading of this new root system made up of the Administration on Aging, the state agencies on aging, area agencies on aging, providers, advisory bodies, and their constituencies.

If we examine the recent developments of a single state (Pennsylvania) over the past three years, the trend in organizational development becomes clear. The state unit on aging has been elevated to a higher status, and the staff complement increased from 12 to 70. The General Assembly has created special committees on aging in both houses. Both houses are seriously considering legislation that would provide a statutory base for the state agency, for the area agencies, and for mandated services. The governor has appointed a Special Assistant for the Aging to coordinate interdepartmental activities. Forty-seven area agencies have been established under the auspices of county governments. Over 400 centers or neighborhood sites have been created. Over 1,000 citizens participate in the advisory committees of the state unit on aging and the area agencies. Each of the centers and neighborhood sites also has an advisory committee.

The Pennsylvania Association of Older People, which recently joined the National Council of Senior Citizens, boasts a membership of 30,000. In Philadelphia the Action Alliance represents a coalition of 150 clubs and centers. Northeastern Pennsylvania now hosts the Federation of Senior Clubs and Center Organizations. The National Caucus on Black Aged has assisted in the establishment of the Pennsylvania Council of Elders. The governor has established a revitalized State Advisory Committee on Aging and four Regional Councils on Aging. We are beginning to observe the development of organizations such as associations of area agency administrators, and associations of center directors.

The above organizations are the rudimentary mechanism of full participation for the aged in our society—the infrastructure that will connect needs and wants with legislative and executive policy makers. To some extent the Pennsylvania experience is being replicated around the nation. It is what Hobart Jackson calls "the emerging network."

Demonstration and Model Building Under the Act.   In addition to the establishment of the Administration on Aging within HEW, the original Older Americans Act provided for the establishment of state agencies on aging and authorized those agencies to make grants to communities for planning and service development. States were permitted wide latitude in establishing and designating agencies. Some were created as independent commissions, others became minor line agencies in existing executive departments. A few were set up as units in the governor's office. No particular pattern has emerged to this day. The placement and purpose of state agencies on aging within state government is constantly changing.

The resources made available to the states for planning and services development in 1965 were modest by any standard. These funds were certainly not sufficient to induce the states to make major investments and commitments on behalf of the aging. As late as 1969 the total national investment for state budgets in planning was $3,218,815, of which only $1,729,434 represented federal costs. Resources for community services and planning were equally modest. The total appropriation under the Older Americans Act was $7,500,000 in 1966 and only $23,000,000 as late as 1969 (Binstock, 1971).

The developmental and experimental nature of the initial program is further emphasized by the fiscal constraints placed on the states in the administration of the grants programs. Until 1973 states were not allowed to make payments to projects that exceeded 75 percent of project costs the first year, 60 percent the second, and 50 percent the third. Until 1969 no support could be provided after the third year. This rule is in stark contrast to the development of Medicare and Medicaid programs, the service titles of the Social Security Act, and other social legislation (U.S. Department of Health, Education and Welfare, 1976).

Even so, the grant-in-aid program provided the first basis for developing experience in community services for the aging. Many of the revisions in the act have been based on the earlier experience. The 1973 Comprehensive Services Amendments, strengthening the state agencies, required the development of local area agencies and the preparation of annual area plans. Moreover, the addition of the Title VII nutrition program can be directly attributed to the early experiences under the act.

Over the years, the lack of clear congressional support tended to retard development and to divert attention from planning and development to agency survival. One respondent observed that

Table 9.2   Annual Budgetary Authorizations Under the Older Americans
Act of 1965, 1966–1977

1966	$ 7,500,000
1967	10,275,000
1968	18,450,000
1969	23,000,000
1970	28,360,000
1971	33,650,000
1972	101,700,000
1973	213,000,012
1974	217,800,000
1975	262,400,000
1976	552,185,000
1977	567,000,000

Source: U.S. Senate Special Committee on Aging (1973; 1976).

survival was such a paramount issue for state units on aging that
they lost sight of the real purpose of the act. State agencies, in
this view, settled for the chance to serve as weak advocates, and
long-run objectives were not formulated.

Observations on the First 10 Years. Precise data are not
readily available to permit any kind of conclusive judgments
about the first 10 years under the act. As a partial substitute,
observations of respondents provide a useful perspective from
which future projections can be made. One respondent con-

tended that the Act has been a great disappointment: "It has been too little too late. . . . It is less than we expected." Another suggested just the opposite. "As historians our expectations were extraordinarily naive. All things considered, I don't think anyone foresaw in March of 1965 what has been achieved in 1976." Yet a third respondent noted that one of the problems in evaluating performance under the act is the evolution of the act itself. The frequent amendments may have so distorted the original objectives of the act that evaluation has to be fixed to precise aspects of the program being administered under the act.

In general, the following observations can be made about the first 10 years under the Older Americans Act of 1965:

First, the act survived. Other programs initiated during the mid-60s have not, most notably the programs initiated under the Economic Opportunity Act. The act survived a direct threat during the early years of the Nixon Administration. The subsequent amendments, especially the addition of Title VII, and the dramatic face-lifting of Title III in 1973, have improved and strengthened it.

Second, the requisite infrastructure is developing. The network of agencies on aging is expanding and taking root. Without presupposing any final judgments, one can cite the fact that in less than three years since the 1973 amendments, nearly 600 local area agencies had been established.

Third, in recent years there has been a trend away from planning and toward services development, away from a state and federal focus and toward a local developmental focus, and away from traditional project funding and toward agency and community-wide programming.

Fourth, although our expectation for a strong agency presence at the federal level is not being achieved through the Administration on Aging, it is being achieved as national organizations like the National Council of Senior Citizens, National Council on Aging, and American Association of Retired Persons expand their influence.

Fifth, the concept of centering influence and authority in a single federal agency and/or a single state agency is not likely to succeed and is not appropriate given the pluralistic nature of our society and our governmental institutions. Title I is not a mandate to state agencies. It is rather a political statement by the Congress that it regards these problems as legitimate public business. Various reports have attempted to digest public benefits available to the elderly. Invariably, these compendia include virtually every agency of state and federal governments. If one examines Title I in terms of broad governmental performance as opposed to performance of a "single federal agency" or a "single state agency," it is possible to record considerable improvements in benefits for older people over the past 10 years.

Sixth, a major criticism of the specific provisions of the Older Americans Act by all respondents was the total inadequacy of the resources base. The enormous gap between the expectations and the limited capacity it has provided to state area agencies jeopardizes the goals of the act and threatens the standing of the agencies. The resource base has not been large enough to encourage much responsiveness from the states. In most instances, the states simply "host" state agencies. In general, services for the aging have not yet become a political issue at the state level. Very few state agencies on aging participate significantly in the state budgetary processes.

CHANGES EXPECTED IN THE NEAR FUTURE (1977–1992)

Viewing the next 15 years as an intermediate period of development has several advantages. It reduces the impact of the rigorous year-to-year conflicts over presidential budgets and congressional appropriations and permits us to observe important trends and directions. It places those conflicts in the broader perspective of planned social change, and relates more realistically to the normal pace of social change in America.

There is a tendency to criticize agencies and programs when in fact the fault is one of national goals and national will. At the national, the state, and the local level, can we develop a consensus on what ought to be the objectives over the next 15 years?

Can enough political influence be mustered to prevail upon the executive and legislative branches of government to provide the leadership, the programs, and the resources to establish a decent way of life for older people in America?

Three factors are necessary to the successful management of change during the next 15 years.

- Public attitudes toward older people must be favorable.
- The need for a more precise definition of service needs and an improved knowledge base must be met.
- Uncertainties about national goals in the context of the new scarcities must be resolved.

Public Attitudes and Political Action. One senses, and the National Council on Aging Harris Poll confirms, an increased public consciousness of the presence and needs of older people (National Council on Aging, 1975). Some observers expressed optimism because this new awareness treats older people universally. It makes no distinction between the elderly poor and nonpoor. The survival of the Older Americans Act may be attributed to its focus on a whole class of people with which the public has developed a new affinity. The current conflict over the Title XX social services eligibility determination procedures may be a preliminary legislative struggle over universality in benefit programs for older people. Older people have become a legitimate political constituency.

The view that "senior power" is of little political use may be short-sighted. Senior power must be understood not simply in political terms, but in social terms. It involves a political foray—but it is also a social foray—into consciousness raising among older people and about older people. It draws support from secondary constituencies. The family tends to vote for politicians who support legislation to help the elderly. With increased expenditures in social benefit programs for older people, an entire system of service providers also "votes aging." Many nonelderly perceive themselves as sharing the goals of improving life for old people.

Pennsylvania, in an otherwise conservative mood, voted 3.5 to 1 in support of a $100,000,000 bond issue to provide low-interest loans for the upgrading of Pennsylvania nursing homes. More recently, in the face of impending budgetary deficits, the Pennsylvania General Assembly approved legislation which guaranteed that all federal increases in SSI benefits will be passed on to the recipients regardless of the level of state supplementation. The survival of the Older Americans Act, and the modest improvements in income benefits, reflect the same interests on the national level. The political effectiveness of senior power must be understood not as the specific development of older people as a unified voting block, but in terms of the value placed on aging issues by a broad spectrum of voters.

Redefining Services Needs and Service Models. We have noted a new trend away from planning and toward services. There are now enough data to establish social service need indicators which would provide new policy options for the development of services programs. Definitions of need based on indicators such as disability, aloneness, advanced age, and low income would help determine what social services should be provided and the extent of public responsibility for such services. It also would help to clarify the scope and scale of problems, permitting the design of integrated services systems to provide a full continuum of care (Benedict & Hoke, 1972).

Increasingly, social service analysts are calling for the establishment of a fundamental conceptual base for the organization and delivery of services. The assumption is that the problems of older people which lead to dependency are developmental. If, during their initial contact, social service providers could use client need indicators to screen clients for specific social service needs, such needs would receive prompt attention, would be prevented from becoming aggravated, and thus would be held at a relatively low level. Such a prescription should presume universal entitlement while limiting provision to those persons who are determined to be "service needy," even though needs will be left unmet and some persons uncared for. This is the impact of all policy decisions in human services and it is appropriate that choices be purposively selective and directed to meeting severe needs first (Benedict & Hoke, 1976).

The development of a conceptual base for comprehensive community-based social services should stem from the desire to maintain older people in the home and in the community. There is a hierarchy of needs which if unmet can lead to dependency. Margaret Blenkner (1969) has called these needs the "normal dependencies" of old age. Such needs become progressively greater with age, and the pattern of dependency is therefore predictable. Service development must recognize the individual, the home, the neighborhood, and the community as the primary bases for organizing and providing comprehensive services. These factors ought to be weighed heavily in the development of service delivery models over the next few years.

Fixing Objectives for the Next 15 Years (1977–1992). The character of state agencies on aging and area agencies on aging has been determined as much by the implementation strategy and the expectations of the Administration on Aging as by congressional intent. In considering change, it is strategic to pay attention to a brief range of mechanisms of change, including legislation and the impact made by professionalization of manpower. The changes that would be useful in the short run would provide a level of financial resources which state agencies and area agencies need to carry out their original purposes. The central idea behind the creation of local agencies was that such agencies should control the financial and other resources, and that this control would place them in a strong negotiation and management position within the community. This has not yet become a reality.

Generally, the respondents' recommendations on future changes fell into five main areas.

1. The functions of state agencies and area agencies should be redefined to encompass service consolidation and delivery rather than loose planning and coordination.
2. State agencies on aging should be strengthened.

3. An adequate resource base for services should be developed.

4. The manpower resource base for aging programs should be improved.

5. Social services should be interfaced with long-term care services.

Redefining the Functions of State and Area Agencies. The need to redefine state agencies and area agencies stems from the fundamental dichotomy posed by the Older Americans Act itself. Two distinct strategies have developed around the country. One focuses on the agencies' function as basic planning agencies, the other stresses the comprehensive development of community-based services. These are distinctly different orientations which, over the long run, will cause severe conflict in the long-range national planning and development of services for the aging. The former is based on the separation of planning from services, and the latter is based on planning as a function of integrated service development. The former is based on knowledge building, and the latter on service development. The former is organized around regionalism, the latter around local communities and neighborhoods. The basic conceptual foundation of each is different. Although there may be some specialized service delivery from a planning base and some planning from a service base, planning organizations and service organizations cannot be equated. They rely on totally different assumptions about needs and the availability of adequate supplies of services.

The circumstances that led to the conceptualization of state and local aging agencies were fundamentally different from those that led, for example, to the conceptualization of regional health planning. In the former case the problem was the total absence of services and service systems; in the latter the problem was primarily one of distribution. The planning model is thus inadequate for dealing with the service problem which confronts this country.

The role and purposes of area agencies should be redefined to encourage their further development as community-based service agencies which function under the aegis of local governments. Decentralization of program administration is an urgent need, and local public accountability should be clearly established. As local public agencies, the area agencies should provide community presence and should be more accessible to the consuming public. To develop statewide and comprehensive services for older people, area agencies need the fundamental long-term underpinning of a state statutory base. As services become more precisely defined, questions of licensure, regulation, and certification will become commonplace. More precise definition of services would increase state and local responsibility in the development of comprehensive services for the aging. It would establish a commitment to provide appropriate resources and authority. It will provide a clear mandate and a base in the community, encouraging cooperation between staff, advisory bodies, centers, service providers, and consumers. It will require the consolidation of responsibility for service development which is now diffused and fragmented under the Older Americans Act, the Social Security Act, revenue sharing, and the Economic Opportunity Act.

The national implications of choosing between the planning model and the service model are considerable. The service model will require a substantial reorganization of the area agency system. Moving toward a comprehensive service strategy will also require that 600 (predominantly) planning organizations be converted into 2000–2500 comprehensive service-oriented area agencies. It will require substantial amendments to several distinct statutes. In spite of this, it is the only responsible course of action.

Developing the State Agencies on Aging. The future concerns of state agencies on aging will revolve around their role and purpose, authority, capacity, and resources. Indications are that in order for state agencies to carry out their responsibilities effectively, these four issues will demand considerable attention over the next few years. State agencies on aging, like area agencies, have been assigned two basic functions: the development and administration of a statewide system of comprehensive community-based services, and the development of state level compre-hensive planning. These responsibilities are distinct and not always compatible.

State agency executives must develop political support if they are to have any effective influence on programs under the juris-diction of other agencies. With a few exceptions, they have not been successful in this effort. National policy will have to focus on extending control of such programs to state agencies. The leadership will have to come from the Congress, because service programs administered by the state are generally established under congressional authority. The administering state and fed-eral agencies will have little or no interest in seeking such changes.

As the functions of state agencies are clarified, the Congress will find it necessary to create greater incentives to change. It may be necessary to extend this principle by requiring state legisla-tures to enact broad legislation to establish a fundamental state statutory base for aging programs as well as authority to consoli-date and reorganize within state governments. Having decided to provide services through states, the entire national strategy for adequately serving older people rests on the states' performance.

Allocating Sufficient Resources.   The problem of develop-ing sufficient resources for services to the aging will persist into the future. This problem is directly related to both of the issues discussed above. The resources requirement is a function of so-cial goals and the definition of needs. When the demographic changes and current estimates of the need for services for the elderly are taken into consideration, we see that creating a re-source base sturdy enough to support comprehensive commu-nity services for older people will require between four and five billion dollars annually.

About 15 percent of the noninstitutionalized older persons over 65 (3,500,000 persons) suffer from disabilities and need special assistance to function normally in the community. This need is exclusive of basic housing costs, institutional health care costs, and income transfers. It presumes a narrow scope of ser-vices and a concentration of services on those defined as service-needy. The current national outlay of less than $500 million dollars annually for services under the Older Americans Act represents only 10 percent of the required sum.

The problem of financing services is predominantly public and predominantly federal. Part of these costs can be met by reordering existing resources such as Titles XVIII, XIX, and XX of the Social Security Act. Expanding services to this level will not reduce the current real costs of long-term care. It may, however, slow the rate of increase in long-term care expenditures, and it may build a base of alternative supports because it will entitle a larger population to basic services.

Developing Adequate Manpower. The expansion and development of services for the elderly that is projected above will require a parallel development of applied social research and educational programs in our colleges and universities. Assuming a trend toward comprehensive services and a gradual transition to a network of 2,000 to 2,500 comprehensive service agencies, and assuming that the resource base nears an adequate level over the next 15 years, it is possible to project a need for a skilled manpower pool of at least 125,000 employees in the primary system of area agencies. In the extended system of community services providers, an additional 600,000 direct service professional and paraprofessional employees will be needed.

The ideal area agency would then serve a total population area of slightly more than 100,000 people, of which 11,000 to 14,000 would be over 65 years. A minimum of 1,600 to 2,000 of these would be noninstitutionalized elderly persons with disabilities serious enough to require personal, social, and health-related services. This ideal agency would require an average professional staff of at least 50 persons, including administrators, planners, service managers, caseworkers, protective service workers, and special service managers. It would also require an expansion of in-home services, transportation services, day care services and legal services, which would add at least 240 to 260 trained workers in each service area (Table 9.3).

Our colleges and universities have not focused their energies on providing the training and education required to produce and

Table 9.3 Average Projections for 2500 Area Agencies on Aging

Service area	100,000
Elderly population 65+	11,000 - 14,000
Non-institutionalized disabled elderly	1,600 - 2,000
AAA professional staff	50 - 60
Service staff	240 - 260
Program budget	$2,000,000

maintain a skilled manpower pool of this magnitude. Coupled with the emerging manpower needs in specialized housing, skilled and intermediate care, and related health services, it is apparent that there is an urgent need for a national manpower policy which realistically addresses these needs.

It is well within our national tradition to utilize the higher education system as a network for fundamental social change. Our social commitment to human services has lacked the kind of vision and direction that encouraged the development of land grant colleges, agricultural extension services, law schools, medical schools, and the public education system.

If the Older Americans Act is to be the primary vehicle for developing comprehensive services, it will have to be amended to ensure the development of an adequate manpower pool in the field. First, education and training goals will need to relate more specifically to the particular needs of the developing system. The focus must shift from aging as a general field of inquiry to aging as a field of practice. Second, education and training standards will need to be imposed upon service agencies as a condition of licensure. Third, incentives will have to be provided to encourage our higher education system to develop instructional programs specific to the field. The emerging system will be only as competent as the people it attracts, because human services are manpower-intensive. Therefore any development of service capability will require the parallel development of manpower resources.

Developing Alternatives to Long-term Care. A fundamental social policy issue of the future is the examination of the role of nursing homes as the sole providers of long-term care. The growth of institutional long-term care cannot be controlled without alternative comprehensive community-based services. Resources should be diverted to a single long-term care system providing a coordinated approach to the needs of the chronically ill elderly rather than two separate but unequal systems of care for the institutionalized and those at home. This means an integration of the management and delivery of skilled and intermediate nursing home care, home health services, and social services.

Many major policies will require modification over the next decade to permit effective interfacing between community and institutional services. Congress should:

- Relax the requirements for "skilled" nursing under Medicare home health regulations to allow for a wider range of nonmedical treatment services which may be more appropriate for the chronically ill elderly.
- Reimburse nonmedical in-home personal care services under Medicare and Medicaid as part of a planned program of long-term services to the chronically ill elderly. (Perhaps the terms Medicare and Medicaid are inappropriate for the broadened service concept.)
- Establish a single set of regulations and a single certification and survey process for home health and other services for the chronically ill elderly under Medicare and Medicaid.
- Direct education, training, and manpower resources into a planned effort to provide the manpower resources needed for a comprehensive long-term services system.
- Legislate a Patients Bill of Rights which supports the right to the least restrictive form of care.
- Provide incentives in Title XIX reimbursement for nursing homes to develop strong rehabilitation programs and to allow continuation of Medicaid payment to maintain care for patients returned to the community, up to the level of payment to the nursing home *or* according to the level of disability—whichever is less.
- Define a program of long-term services reimbursable by the level of disability based on cost of service, regardless of the setting in which the service is provided.
- Build a capacity at the local level to manage multiple funds and complex service needs. Payment should be channeled through a long-term service management organization (perhaps area agencies on aging) which can supervise the provision of a total range of services in or out of institutions.

These actions would move toward eliminating the distinction between social and health services, and would create incentives more in keeping with consumer concerns. Community-based management of all long-term services would be required, but this is completely compatible with the national goal of normalization of living arrangements and deinstitutionalization. It is also consistent with the development of area agencies as comprehensive community services agencies.

OPTIONS FOR THE MORE DISTANT FUTURE: THE OLDER AMERICANS ACT IN 2025

Over the long run, we can anticipate a continuing evolutionary trend for the Older Americans Act. Few perceive the future for older people simply in terms of the act. Most observers suggest that center stage will be occupied by the maintenance and improvement of Social Security Act benefit programs. One respondent suggested that the gradual extension of SSA into some minor service areas might lead to the consolidation of the AoA and the SSA systems.

It appears that in the long run, as the income maintenance system, the health system, and the social services system expand, they are likely to converge. The key question is whether each will remain a separate and distinct system or whether, as a result of policy or pure political influence, one system will prevail.

Recent economic difficulties and resource scarcities make it clear that the continued improvement of human services will require major new sacrifices. Achieving a state of well-being for the aged cannot rest on the residual benefits of an ever expanding economy. It will require a redistribution of existing national resources. Only the most concerted advocacy will succeed in protecting the fragile services network, because the thrust of the future may be retrenchment.

One respondent raised a new and troubling problem: the continued decline in the quality of life of our core cities is creating a new dependency problem—not of classes of people, but of whole places. He suggests that if national policy does not reconstruct the social and economic base of core cities in the immediate future, we will have massive "refugee problems" even before 2025. The cities may become repositories for the poor, the elderly, and the maladjusted. He raises the question of the relevance of social policies which do not address this overwhelming issue, and suggests that policy research on the status of older people in urban settings is urgently required. As a result, it may be necessary to create "islands of safety" for older people in the cities or to relocate them to a more secure, less troubled environment.

The sheer size of the older population and the related demand for health and welfare services will keep older people on the public agenda for the foreseeable future. The clients of the service system of the future will be clearly distinguishable because future cohorts of older persons will revolutionize the image of late life. They will be educated, vigorous, and socially involved. The service needs of those who are disabled and socially dependent will thus be even more pronounced and distinct than they are today. This may provide the impetus for narrowing the focus of the act to the single mission of developing comprehensive community services for the functionally disabled aged.

Basic income transfers will not alleviate the need for an Administration on Aging and the Older Americans Act. There will also be an ongoing need to assess the impact of current policies on the development of future systems. How will improvements in pension benefits affect Social Security benefit structures over the long run? How solvent are those pension systems? What will be the impact of national health insurance on the design and development of social services programs?

Projections of the next 50 years must be highly speculative. The recent history of human services does not offer any firm clues, and the pace of change imposes severe limitations. There are many volatile issues which will impinge on long-term social developments. Nonetheless, one senses cautious optimism, and a general, if slow, trend toward improvements in those human service systems that affect the quality of life for future generations of older people.

REFERENCES

Benedict, R., & Hoke, R. Caring for elderly persons, Harrisburg, Unpublished Report, 1973.

Benedict, R., & Hoke, R. Toward community services for the aging: A state agency perspective. In G. Maddox (Ed.), *Planning services for older people: Translating objectives into effective programs.* Durham, N.C.: Duke University Press, 1976.

Binstock, R. *Planning: Background and issues.* Washington, D.C.: U.S. Government Printing Office, 1971.

Blenkner, M. Normal dependencies of aging. *Occasional Papers in Gerontology,* No. 6. Ann Arbor: University of Michigan Press, 1969.

Brotman, H. B. Who are the aged: A demographic view. *Occasional Papers in Gerontology,* No. 1. Ann Arbor: University of Michigan Press, 1968.

National Center for Health Statistics. *Chronic conditions and limitations of activity and mobility, United States—July 1965–June 1967.* Data from the National Health Survey. Series 10, No. 61. Rockville, Maryland: National Center for Health Statistics, U.S. Department of Health, Education and Welfare, 1971.

National Council on the Aging. *The myth and reality of aging in America.* Washington, D.C.: National Council on the Aging, 1975.

U.S. Bureau of the Census. *Census of population: 1970, general population characteristics.* Final report PC(1)-B40. Washington, D.C.: U.S. Government Printing Office, 1970.

U.S. Department of Health, Education and Welfare. *Older Americans Act of 1965, as amended.* Washington, D.C.: U.S. Government Printing Office, 1976.

U.S. Senate Committee on Aging. *Older Americans comprehensive services amendments of 1973.* Washington, D.C.: U.S. Government Printing Office, 1973.

U.S. Senate Special Committee on Aging. *Action on aging in the 94th Congress.* Washington, D.C.: U.S. Government Printing Office, 1976.

White House Conference on Aging, 1961. *The nation and its older people.* Washington, D.C.: U.S. Government Printing Office, 1961.

-Part V-

CONCLUSION

Providing Income and Opportunities for Work: Future Policy Choices

Barbara Rieman Herzog

Current Climate of Opinion. After a decade of self-congratulation that at last, with Medicare and higher Social Security benefits in place, the nation is finally beginning to provide decently for its elderly population, the country's mood has changed. Within a single three-week period in early 1977, all major national TV networks ran special reports on aging, and the press was full of articles on the general theme of "the graying of America." The focus of these stories was on demographic change and on the impact of growing numbers of elderly upon the nation's pocketbook. As *Newsweek* (February 28, 1977) put it, the most clear-cut question posed by the projections is "How will the nation bear the cost of caring for so many old people?"

The changed focus has been precipitated by the press, which finally began to notice in 1976 that the Social Security system was no longer taking in enough money to keep up with its obligations, and that, anticipating payroll tax increases, some cities were thinking of opting out of Social Security. A little homework by the press revealed that for several years, the Social Security Administration, the Senate Committee on Aging, and other experts had been well aware that demographic change and economic downturn were going to necessitate either changes in benefits, payroll tax increases, or both. By 1976, politicians too began to take note that the future was going to be more expensive than the past. Former Secretary of the Treasury William Simon said he had looked into the state of the Social Security program and had found it "shocking." Meanwhile, Social Security officials responded to the sudden alarm by issuing statements admitting that yes, some changes would have to be made, but that the system was very much solvent and that all retirees would get their proper benefits.

The issue didn't go away, however. Once future demographic projections became common knowledge, people began applying them to other areas and began to recognize that the costs of company and union pensions, public employee pensions, military pensions, and health care for the elderly will all rise sharply over the next half century. Along with the calculations came the first public rumblings that perhaps future benefits should be cut back rather than increased.

Future Needs of the Elderly.   If all of our elderly population enjoyed even a minimal state of well-being, these rumblings would not be so disturbing. Unfortunately, this is not the case. A long catalogue of unattended ills is inappropriate here, but a short review of a few income-related problems may offer some perspective.

Too many older people still live in grinding poverty—fully 15 percent in 1976, according to the usual Census Bureau calculations (Brotman, 1977). The Congressional Budget Office has recently (1977) recalculated the figure, arriving at only four percent, but this figure counts all government assistance, including Medicare and Medicaid, as income. Without inclusion of health benefits as income, the CBO study indicates that 10.5 percent are in poverty. However, considering Medicare and Medicaid payments as "normal" income seems unjustified in view of the fact that older people require more medical attention than younger people, unless the poverty level for older people is also raised to reflect their greater expenditures on health care. Another problem with the CBO study is that it is based on estimates rather than hard data as to who actually received medical benefits (U.S. Senate, Special Committee on Aging, 1976).

In any case the official poverty level is set at an incredibly low figure: $2,572 for an elderly individual and $3,232 for an elderly couple in 1975. These figures are over a thousand dollars *lower* than the Bureau of Labor Statistics' low-income budget, which allows only $27.40 per week for food and $3.81 per week for clothing—*per couple* (U.S. Department of Labor, 1976). One might wonder whether the poverty level has not been left at this extremely low level so as to salve our national conscience. Raising it to a more realistic level would define many more as living in poverty. At present—as low as it is—36 percent of blacks and 33 percent of persons of Spanish origin fall below it (U.S. DHEW, 1977), and a quarter of all widows live in poverty (U.S. DHEW, 1976).

The poor elderly are not the only segment of the older population for whom America has not yet made adequate provision. Many older people on the other end of the income spectrum feel deprived in a different way: because they have been mandatorily retired, or because they can't find work. Clearly, many older people prefer to retire from the often disagreeable jobs which society provides. But many would like to keep working, at least part-time, at the same or different jobs. The 1974 Harris Poll found that 31 percent of people 65 and over who were retired or unemployed would like to be working. Our failure to provide employment opportunities has meant a loss of well-being for the many who are well enough to work.

Apart from the existence of too many poor elderly, and too many who want jobs but cannot find them, major problems of health care and services remain to be solved. Our nursing home problem—a complex issue comprised of elements ranging from tender loving greed to inadequate Medicaid financing—is not close to solution. Almost all of us would prefer our own homes to nursing homes, yet the services making this possible are woefully inadequate. In the U.S. there is one home health aide for every 5,000 elderly persons; Great Britain has one for every 750 (Maddox, 1976). Other services to facilitate independent living

—transportation, shopping, home repair, telephone reassurance —have been initiated in many cities but are still so limited that they can serve only a small proportion of those who need them. The economic problems should not be overstated. Whatever their difficulties with status or roles, many older people have an adequate income. Continuing to increase real benefits and income for all elderly, regardless of income, may not be among our future priorities. However demographic pressures and the prospect of higher dependency costs should not keep us from improving benefits for the many who still have inadequate incomes and cannot afford, or cannot find, adequate care and social services.

Past Mistakes. As a society we have spent not inconsiderable sums of tax dollars to improve life for the elderly. Apart from the simple need to spend more, why are we not further along in providing a decent quality of life for the older population?

One answer is the rapid increase in the numbers of elderly. But the problems we face today are caused less by an oversupply of older people than by an undersupply of economic savvy and political will. Over the past decade, had we had the will to create a healthier economy and solve our chronic unemployment problems, the policy of abrupt and full retirement at 65 or earlier would probably not have become so widespread. Instead, the barriers to part-time work would have been reduced, jobs might have been redesigned to make them more agreeable, and job retraining would have been made more available to older workers. Had our economy been healthier, older people would probably have had a greater range of options—scaling down to part-time work (which would have been plentiful, not scarce) with partial pensions; continuing to work in new, less demanding, or simply different jobs for which they would have been retrained by the government or employers; continuing to work in their regular jobs, which might have been redesigned to make them more attractive; or retiring early with disability pay were they too ill to work. Money saved by not providing full retirement to everyone at 65 or earlier could have been spent to raise the standard of living of the poor, and to provide adequate nursing and home care services for the frail and ill elderly.

In short, our society would have retained more of the characteristics of traditional societies where, as people grew old, they shifted to work which was somewhat less demanding physically but not necessarily less demanding mentally, and finally, when they became dependent, received good care.

Hindsight is cheap, and the above factors were certainly not the only ones which led to our current situation. Moreover, just because people are now beginning to worry whether we can afford the future costs of support for the elderly does not mean we cannot afford such costs. Europeans tax themselves at a much higher rate for their social welfare services than we do. And, as Clark and Spengler have shown in Chapter 2, the future cost of support of both old people and children *combined* will probably rise only a relatively modest amount, assuming that current support levels remain constant.

Even if it involves increased redistribution of income, we should be willing to maintain and where necessary improve the elderly's standard of living. But will there be sufficient political support to allow this? What factors will most influence costs, and the extent to which future taxpayers will be willing to pay those costs?

Impact of Economic Conditions on Future Support for the Elderly. Even if one is reasonably optimistic about the future, some areas of uncertainty must be acknowledged, including the possibility of growing intergenerational bitterness and partial repudiation of promised benefits. Much depends on the state of the economy. If real wages are not increasing, working people may come to resent the leisure and income which their tax dollars help provide for the elderly. In hard times, ads showing healthy, tanned retirees basking in the sun, and benefits like subsidized bus fares may cause a voter reaction against maintaining promised levels of support. Impoverished old people in dingy rooming houses are much less visible than are affluent retirees.

EFFECT ON SOCIAL SECURITY AND PUBLIC PENSIONS. If times are reasonably good, tax increases necessary to maintain or improve benefits for the elderly will probably not seem too onerous. Now that, for example, Social Security's overindexing problem is corrected, Munnell calculates in Chapter 5 that the payroll tax rate required to finance current levels of benefits in the year 2050 would rise to 19.2 percent. If part of this amount were shifted to general revenue financing, so that the bite would not be as obvious or as regressive, this increase over a 70-year period seems tolerable. Economic conditions will also have an impact upon the acceptability of taxation to meet public employee pension costs. Given increased numbers of older people and the largely unfunded condition of many city and state pension systems, local taxes will have to be increased to cover these obligations. If personal income is not also increasing, the bite will feel bigger.

EFFECT ON PRIVATE PENSIONS. The economic health of the nation will also affect the political and economic viability of support for the elderly in another area: private pensions, where costs are rapidly increasing. At General Motors, for example, the pension bill has doubled in the last decade and will double again in the next 10 to 15 years (*Newsweek,* February 28, 1977). Although private pensions are better funded than most state and local pensions, many companies have huge unfunded liabilities and make risky assumptions. The ability of employers to meet their pension promises depends on the soundness of their estimates of how much must be invested each year, and on whether the investments produce the expected returns. If actuarial estimates are incorrect because inflation is higher than anticipated, and/or the economy is depressed, investment returns may fall short of expectations. Under the 1974 ERISA reforms, a company is obligated to dip far into its corporate assets (up to 30 percent of net worth) to meet its pension promises. One can envision that in bad times, this might drive some companies into bankruptcy. Were this to happen on a small scale, the Pension Benefit Guarantee Corporation (PBGC) could cover indebtedness. On a larger scale such bankruptcies would obviously result in severe dislocations, to say nothing of exceeding PBGC resources.

Impact of Prolongation of Life. The projections in this book are all based on the assumption that no dramatic longevity breakthroughs will occur, but rather that the number of years which people live will continue to increase gradually. Within the last decade, longevity has increased just a bit faster than predicted. According to demographers at the Social Security Administration, life expectancy projections are even now being slightly revised upward. These minor revisions will make almost no difference in the projections described in this book. If, however, a major medical breakthrough should occur, and the average life expectancy were extended by 10 or more years over the next half century, our projections would be less than helpful, and the costs of maintaining present benefit levels would soar.

Breakthroughs are by definition hard to predict, and not surprisingly, most scientists do not foresee any major ones in the near future. Albert Rosenfeld's recent book (1976) entitled *Prolongevity* discusses the progress being made by scientists who are studying the causes of aging and how longevity can be increased. After discussions with many prominent scientists, Rosenfeld's best guess is that "with a bit of good luck and not too much bad luck, modest breakthroughs will begin to occur within a few decades" (p. 125). On the other hand, there is at least a possibility that deaths from environmentally caused cancers may be on the increase. In any case, it should be recognized that the Census Department's projections may be wrong because of misestimates of either fertility or mortality, and that resultant support costs may turn out to be higher than anticipated.

Impact of Changes in the Average Age of Retirement. In addition to the state of the economy and the average lifespan, the average age of retirement will have a great effect on costs of providing for the elderly population. If everyone chose—or was forced—to retire at 55, projected support costs would rise dramatically. Given the substantial possibility that the economy will not be as healthy as we would like, or that we are fortunate enough to reduce the death rate from diseases of old age, it would behoove us to pay close attention to the average age of retirement and to prevent or reverse its further decline, except perhaps in a few disagreeable or dangerous occupations. At a time when there is some danger of polarization between the workers and retirees, and when future refusal by the former to adequately support the latter is a possibility, it does not make sense to increase the dependency burden by further lowering the average age of retirement. On the contrary, the next thirty years —before the elderly population bulge occurs in 2010—is the appropriate time to adopt policies halting or reversing this risky trend.

Prospects for the Future. The authors of this book have offered a number of suggestions aimed at intelligent planning for change in the policies and programs affecting the income of the elderly. The following pages provide an overall perspective on the major issues and possibilities in the areas of income-in-kind, pensions, Social Security, and income from work.

PROVISION OF HEALTH CARE SERVICES

Unmet—and overmet—needs. It is all too clear that we have not yet resolved the question of how to provide adequate health care for the older population of this country. The best of intentions have been thwarted by (most conspicuously) the rapid inflation of health care costs and (less conspicuously) the failure to provide integrated health and social services. The result has been that although costs of Medicare have skyrocketed, by 1976 the program was paying only 38 percent of the medical expenses of the average older person (U.S. Senate Special Committee on Aging, 1976). It is equally unfortunate that older people are too often forced into a total medical and service care setting—the nursing home—when what they would prefer is just enough medical care and social services to allow them to remain at home.

The Design of National Health Insurance. At present, however, debate over health care is focussed not on the needs of the elderly, but on national health insurance. Is it coming, when is it coming, and what form will or should it take? The problems involved in designing a system for all—and particularly in designing one that will be able to hold down costs—are so complex that the issue of improved care for the elderly has been relegated to a back seat. Yet those interested in the welfare of the elderly

cannot simply assume that all of the costly systems currently
under consideration will necessarily entail improved services for
the elderly. In fact, just the reverse may be true. If we create more
demand for a limited supply of health services, the amount available to the elderly may decline, or, depending on the design of
incentives, the elderly could become undesirable patients whose
patronage some providers might try to evade.

The issues currently of most interest to those considering national health insurance appear to include the following:

1. How to control quality (e.g., peer review, national licensure, continuing education, recertification)
2. How to control costs (e.g., price controls, controls on the
   number of hospital beds, prospective and all-inclusive hospital rates, utilization review)
3. How to control uneven distribution of services (e.g., incentives to locate in rural areas or inner cities, creation of a
   national health service corps) (Elwood, 1974)
4. How to structure benefit payments (e.g., to provide for
   medical costs only, or also for costs for homemakers and
   other services).

COST CONTROL. Because of skyrocketing health care costs,
control of costs is currently the most urgent of these issues, and
if we are not careful, could be emphasized to the exclusion of
other equally important areas. The health maintenance organization (HMO) model of care delivery described in Henry Brehm's
article has, as he points out, the potential advantage of very
effectively controlling costs. Payments would not be fees for separate services, but regular stipends for the ongoing care of however many people the HMO had on its rolls. The HMO's
emphasis on prevention is obviously very desirable for the elderly, but one potential drawback does present itself—the possibility of "creaming."

The HMO is provided the incentive to keep people well and
to treat them less often, rather than more. This same incentive
might work to induce some HMOs to seek the healthiest people
to include on their rolls, necessitating as little treatment as possi-

ble and thus keeping the HMO's expense/income ratio as small as possible. Because older people require more health care, it will clearly be necessary to provide a higher rate for elderly enrollees. However, certain HMOs might still try to "cream off" the healthiest older people, providing less than adequate services to the sickest in order to encourage them to transfer to some other HMO. Thus, from the elderly health-care consumer's point of view, the present fee-for-service Medicare reimbursement system might appear to provide more secure care than a system of competing HMOs—unless HMO's incentives are very carefully planned.

Because of the differences in needs, the health care interests of the elderly individual and the interests of the nonelderly may be quite divergent. As George Maddox wrote of health care in the U.K. and the U.S.:

> Medical education and health care delivery systems in both countries were designed to manage acute, not chronic illness; they are therefore mismatched with the particular needs of older persons for preventive, primary and long term care. . . . The mismatch is troublesome in the United Kingdom and dramatic in the United States (Maddox, 1976, p. 2).

Advocates of the elderly must pay considerable attention to ensure that health care proposals provide for the elderly's special needs and do not deprive them of sufficient or proper forms of care in the interest of cost cutting. Likewise, because many elderly people live in rural areas or the inner city, sufficient incentives must be provided to ensure availability of medical services in these "less desirable" areas. Finally, the question of how to expand mental health services must be addressed, so that such services are not ignored in the rush toward a "comprehensive" new system.

INTEGRATION OF HEALTH AND SOCIAL SERVICES. Probably the most basic issue is how to create an efficient and equitable system which takes account of the elderly's special needs for nursing home and home care services as well as hospital services. Few of the proposals for national health insurance fully address the problem of nursing home or at-home care.

One possibility is that health care coverage could provide for all three kinds of care—hospital, at-home, and nursing home—allowing the patient to choose between them, up to a certain maximum cost level. A new arrangement is necessary to stimulate and coordinate the provision of the services needed to enable more people to remain at home (e.g., home health care, transportation, home repair, shopping and telephone reassurance services). In Chapter 9, Robert Benedict suggests that the already established area agencies on aging might perform this function. Other proposals have been set forth, including bills introduced by Representative Barber Conable, which would set up long-term care centers (H.R. 2029, 3144, 3641, and 4006). Another option is to rely on cities to continue developing such programs from their health or welfare departments.

Whatever the resolution, the benefit structure must not, as it now does, encourage hospitalization over the use of nursing homes (through more complete Medicare coverage for hospital than for nursing home care), and the use of nursing homes over the use of at-home services (through overly strict Medicare and Medicaid limitations on at-home services).

Providing good health care for the elderly already costs us a great deal. The more than $1,200 per year which we spend for the health care of an average elderly individual is considerably higher than the amount spent in most European countries (Anderson, 1976). The result, unfortunately, has not been better overall care. Esther Ammundsen's chapter indicates that the European countries have progressed somewhat further than the United States with their integration of health and social services, which may be one reason why their costs are lower and services better. We use more nursing homes; they use more home health and other services.

Understandably, the issue of cost control has assumed center stage at this point in our history. The soaring expenses of the past 10 years have been disheartening, and the prospect of a large increase in the elderly population is making cost control seem all the more urgent. Future policy must limit cost increases due to unwarranted high fees, inappropriate treatment, inefficiencies, or irrational purchase of every new piece of equipment that comes on the market. Yet cost increases (and resulting increased taxes) to expand and improve care may be in the interests of the elderly. If there are to be future trade-offs between higher Social Security benefits and better health care, someone had better poll the elderly to ask which they would prefer.

OPTIONS FOR PUBLIC POLICY ON PRIVATE PENSIONS

Of the various systems affecting the income of the elderly, the private pension system is, as a whole, the least understood. The mechanics of individual pension plans have been well analyzed, but future effects of the pension system on the economy as a whole have received less attention. Peter Drucker's 1976 book, *The Unseen Revolution*, overstates the neglect, as a rebuttal by James Henry (1977) indicates. Nonetheless, Drucker points out many soft spots in our current understanding, and it seems fair to say that the future impact of pensions on the economy, and conversely, their dependence on the state of the economy, remain in serious need of further examination.

Current Trends and Government Leverage. Some experts (including several of the contributors to this book) anticipate an expansion in the role of private pensions. Others have predicted contraction, citing plan terminations since the inception of the 1974 ERISA reform. Trade journals such as *Pension World* and the *Employee Benefit Plan Review* maintain a guardedly optimistic tone, although they are replete with complaints about the difficulties of operating under complex ERISA rules.

What is the optimum mix of private pensions and Social Security, assuming we can achieve the mix we want through government policy? James Schulz (1976, 1977) presents some of the basic factors to be considered. We do not know, however, how easy it will be to bring about the mix we decide is best. If corporate leaders decide that pensions are too costly or destabilizing it may be difficult—and imprudent—for government to prevent cutbacks. Some leverage certainly exists: for instance, in 1977, the government will refrain from taxing $6.5 billion of the wages earmarked for pensions by companies which provide them. (U.S. Senate, Committee on the Budget, 1976). Since offering pensions presumably affords these companies a hiring advantage over companies without pensions (except among those individuals who come to believe an IRA may be more advantageous than a company pension), this subsidy must have an impact on decisions to retain or abandon pension plans, but whether its effect is significant is not clear.

Regardless of the subsidy's current effect, the government's long-run power to regulate is clearly important. How then should the government exercise this leverage? Should it try to induce an increase or a decrease in the role of private pensions? Should it try to change the percentage of the work force covered by such pensions, or how fast vesting occurs, or how and where pension funds are invested?

Would increased coverage by private pensions be beneficial? A possible plan. Suppose, for example, we wanted to explore the policy option of bringing all privately employed persons under private pension coverage. Under one plan to bring this about, the government might refrain from taxing a certain amount of each worker's wage, and require that each firm either invest the money in its own pension fund, or else put it into an IRA account or some kind of quasi-governmental but independent fund, which would invest it for the worker. An employer's former option, the offering of a pension, would thus become a specified duty.

Although such a plan might seem, on its face, an attractive way of expanding private coverage, it would clearly require thorough analysis of the attendant costs and impact on the economy, as well as on various interest groups. The following paragraphs describe some of the questions which would need answers. The questions are listed here both because they shed light on the merits of the above proposal, and because they are the questions that need to be applied to other proposals for changing (or not changing) the private pension system.

Questions that should be asked of any pension proposal.
1. What would be the impact of the resulting pension system upon capital formation? If savings would be increased,

would this be desirable, or would too much forced saving hurt the economy in certain instances? At what point would benefits paid out surpass income paid in, with resultant reduction in capital available for investment? Is the threat of negative capital formation (Drucker, 1976) serious, or can the nation twist other dials (Okun, 1975) to ensure the appropriate level of saving and investment?

2. What would be the effects on investment patterns? Non-institutional investors can afford to take substantial risks for the prospect of substantial gains. In contrast, pension investors are under great pressure to make relatively conservative investments in order to assure that future promises can be met, and because of the 1974 regulation requiring that investments be "prudent." Will this pressure result in a trend toward traditional, "blue chip" investment, and a shortage of venture capital for projects offering the possibility of rapid economic growth, such as alternative energy technologies, etc.? If so, how serious is this?

3. What would be the effects of encouraging private pensions in lieu of expanding Social Security under various assumptions of economic growth? Will plans be able to meet their promises in most instances? If not, what would the effects be? If, under pressure from corporate management, actuaries underestimate future costs and these costs mushroom, will the 30 percent of net worth limitation on liability provide incentive for widespread terminations? What would be the impact on the economy of specified pension arrangements during a period of serious economic decline? Do some arrangements lock us in and deter recovery more than others? Can local pension funds be protected against expropriation by financially desperate city governments?

4. Although the above proposal to increase coverage might seem relatively simple, the mechanics of implementing it would be very complex, and would require a thorough assessment. For example, what kinds of bodies would have charge of investing the funds of workers whose employers do not have plans of their own? The many banks which offer

the IRAs? If so, how good are their disclosure and investment policies? Quasi-public pension trusts? If so, who would control these trusts and where would they invest their funds? Government control of such trusts might be viewed as beneficial by those who prefer more planning in the economy and more government leverage to invigorate a failing sector—such as housing in 1975—by investing in it. Others, more worried about an expanding bureaucracy, might prefer to leave the trusts in private hands. Might we, as Drucker (1976) suggests, establish boards to make pension funds more accountable to their "owners"? Perhaps individuals should have some choice over to whom they entrust their retirement funds, and should be able to decide between a pension fund offered by their employer, an IRA, or a quasi-public pension trust. What would be the implications of allowing such a choice?

5. What would be the effect on the Social Security system? And what would be the relative costs of providing additional coverage via private pensions as opposed to Social Security if costs of regulation and administration were counted?

6. What would be the effect on employers? Under the example proposed above, small businessmen who would be forced to contribute might find that their costs would increase since they might not want to (or be able to) reduce wages by the amount they would be forced to invest for pension purposes. On the other hand, the proposed change might make hiring and retaining workers easier, a factor which might compensate for the required pension contribution.

7. What would be the effect on workers whose employers do not now provide pension plans? Those who already have their own IRA account, and thus are already beneficiaries of a tax subsidy, might see no gains. (The tax subsidy to these individuals—most of whom are professional and other high-income self-employed individuals—will amount to $695 million in 1977) (U.S. Senate, Committee on the Budget, 1976). Those who do not have their own IRA ac-

counts might be better off at retirement time under such a rule, (assuming that whatever group controlled their pension contributions were carefully regulated and able to meet future promises). However they could be somewhat worse off during their working years, since employers might well respond by taking the contribution required by the government directly from their pay.

Need to Assess Pension Impact before Shifting Policy Emphasis from Social Security. Although the above proposal to extend private pension coverage might appear especially attractive in a climate where sentiment is mounting against further Social Security tax increases, a rigorous analysis might reveal that such a proposal would be costly and cumbersome, or generate unpalatable effects on the economy. Quite clearly, without such analysis, adoption of a government-stimulated expansion of the private pension system would certainly be risky.

Fortunately, because our political process is usually such a slow one, all of the interest groups described above would have a chance to express their views about any proposed changes. What is much harder to ensure in evaluating any proposal for change is a sophisticated and reasonably accurate economic prediction of what the change would mean for the economy as a whole.

In any case, Congress is not likely to tackle the question of private pensions again soon, since the energy invested in passing the 1974 ERISA reform depleted enthusiasum for further action (Haneberg, 1977). Only our shaky public employee pensions, which are building up billions of dollars of unfunded promises, are likely to be the subject of much Congressional scrutiny in the near future. We can ill afford to assume, however, that all is well with the private pension system, and that because it has been "reformed" it is a reliable instrument of social and economic policy. The 1974 reformers were more concerned with enhancing individual rights to pensions than with the pension system's effects on the economy and the social structure. There needs to be a harder look at this whole area before we can intelligently decide whether to try to expand the private pension system.

THE FUTURE OF THE SOCIAL SECURITY SYSTEM

Interrelationship with Other Income-Support Programs.
The Social Security system has been subject to much closer scrutiny than have the private and public employee pension systems. We know considerably more about its current effects and future problems, and have a better idea of some of the changes that should be made. For example, the double-indexing problem, which overcompensated future retirees for inflation (see Chapter 5) was in great need of correction. In other areas, however, the best policy choices are less clear, and cannot be intelligently determined without close analysis of future prospects for interrelated programs, including private pensions, health care, and opportunities for work.

For example, a case can be made for stabilizing overall benefit awards under Social Security and increasing coverage and benefit levels under private pensions, as suggested by Francis King in Chapter 6. The public is certainly unhappy about the prospect of substantial increases in Social Security payroll taxes. Moreover, greater reliance on private pensions could reduce the need for a steep tax increase to pay for Social Security benefits when the retiree "bulge" occurs after the year 2010. It is not clear that the working population will think it fair suddenly to have steep tax increases imposed on them at that time. The burden could be spread out by forcing more saving through the funded private pension system over the next 30 years, rather than hoping that workers after 2010 will not rebel and suddenly cut back the pay-as-you-go Social Security benefits.

However the case for stabilizing Social Security and increasing private pensions would seem to hold only under certain conditions:

1. If private pension coverage can be expanded so that more than 43 percent of the nation's workers are covered, and so that more of those covered actually vest and receive benefits.

2. If regulations are successful in preventing willful or inadvertent mismanagement of pension funds.

3. If business continues to find its interests well served by sponsoring pension plans despite strict regulation and in conditions of uncertainty about future inflation.

4. If expansion of pension fund investment is found to be beneficial for the economy as a whole.

Quite possibly, these conditions may not prevail, and the current enthusiasm for trying to shift emphasis from Social Security to private pensions will dwindle. Bearing in mind that the biggest decisions concerning the future of the Social Security system should really not be undertaken without first examining private pension policy, what areas seem most in need of attention at this time?

Areas in Which Social Security Policy Requires Improvement. 1. Since too many older people still live in or near poverty, in coming years emphasis should be placed upon giving these people, sometimes for the first time, a minimally decent standard of living. Through what mechanism should this be accomplished?

MUNNELL PROPOSAL. Alicia Munnell argues in Chapter 5 for shifting the many people now receiving minimum Social Security benefits to SSI, allowing SSI to handle all welfare functions, and leaving Social Security as an insurance program paying proportional benefits. This would have the advantage of preventing the many people who are now collecting both Social Security and other public pensions from receiving unwarranted subsidies in the form of Social Security benefits which are disproportional to the amounts they have paid into the system. However, she does not address the other available remedies for this problem (such as paying only proportional benefits to those with other pensions) and her discussion leaves two questions unanswered:

First, is it in the public interest to require many more people to apply for means-tested, welfare-type SSI benefits rather than to receive redistributed funds automatically as regular Social Security? At present, SSI is still not fully subscribed. Some older people may not know about the program, but others are probably unwilling to apply for the welfare-type benefits even though they would be happy to receive them in the form of an automatic, non-means-tested Social Security check.

Second, do the advantages of her plan outweigh the risk of jeopardizing the redistribution of income which has been a relatively unquestioned part of Social Security? Because SSI is a welfare program, benefits provided under it could be subject to yearly congressional battles, possibly resulting in abrupt reduction of benefits. Although at present Social Security minimum benefits currently serve a welfare function as well as an insurance function, thus far they have been isolated from congressional welfare debates.

CURRENT SYSTEM WITH PARTIAL RELIANCE ON GENERAL REVENUE FINANCING. Another possible way of making payments would be to continue the current system of relying primarily on the Social Security system (including the payment of benefits which are either disproportionately high or low), while using SSI to provide an income floor for the poorest of the elderly. As the need for additional financing increases, additional funds could be obtained from general revenue financing, as former Social Security Commissioner Robert Ball (1976) and many others have suggested.

DEMOGRANT METHOD. There are other, and in my opinion, better, alternatives. Eveline Burns (1965) and others have argued for a basic flat grant to every old person, combined with a Social Security payment program that is proportional to money paid into the system. The flat grant (sometimes called a *demogrant*) would not be subject to a means test, but would be paid to everyone attaining a certain age, and therefore would not have a welfare stigma, as do SSI benefits. Many European countries use such a system, finding it both more progressive and easier to administer than a means-tested minimum payment. The objection can be raised that because the flat grant is not means-tested it will cost the public treasury more money. One partial answer would be to include Social Security payments as income for income tax purposes. Doing so would mean that some (better-off) elderly persons would in effect have to return part of their flat benefit to the Treasury. This would be a partial means test—just as is the income tax itself—but one administered in a less harsh, less stigmatizing manner than are welfare programs such as SSI.

Whichever distribution mechanism is chosen, there should be an aggressive effort to seek out the poor elderly and to make certain that *all* older people, whether or not they have contributed to Social Security, are assured of an income well above the poverty line—which is not yet the case under SSI.

2. Social Security should cover all people who work for a minimum period. This should be true whether or not they work for wages, and thus women ought to be covered in their own right. Although keeping families together is an admirable goal, a housewife ought not be held hostage to her Social Security benefits (which she loses if she is divorced before 10 years). This problem could be remedied without great additional costs since a large number of women already collect spouses' benefits, and the addition of those who currently lose out would not be very expensive. A number of solutions are possible, such as attributing a part of the family wage-earner's salary to the housewife (or househusband). This might be either a percentage or a flat rate. The government might also contribute an amount for women caring for children or frail elderly people. Each individual would thus have his or her own Social Security credits, which would be collectable regardless of marital status. The issue of spouses' benefits, a long-standing sore point with both single people and divorcees, would thus be at least partially resolved in favor of individual benefits.

3. Although correcting the indexing error has reduced the projected cost increases, raising benefits for the poor and providing Social Security credits for at-home spouses would necessitate higher tax increases than those shown in Munnell's projections. Realistically, there is some upper limit on how much future workers will tax themselves to support future retirees. Therefore relying solely upon redistribution from the working population to the elderly to increase benefits for the poorest elderly is not advisable; redistribution among the elderly themselves must also

occur. Income from Social Security should be taxed along with all other income, including income from securities, private pensions, military pensions, or work. Such income taxes should not touch those with incomes near or below the poverty level, and should follow the current pattern of progressively higher rates for higher incomes.

4. Another way of reducing the burden upon the working population would be to raise the age of retirement. Certainly we cannot allow it to fall further. The age at which one can receive Social Security (as opposed to disability payments) may initially have been set too low, and has probably played a role in fostering mandatory retirement practices. Abolition of mandatory retirement at 65 has long been warranted and would receive widespread support from most older people. But mention of raising the retirement age is generally construed to mean raising the age at which Social Security benefits will be paid. Any sudden increase would concentrate the burden of reducing Social Security costs on a small segment of the population: the people who have been wanting to retire, and counting upon being able to do so at a certain time. No matter how desirable the objective of making it possible for people to remain in the labor force longer, it seems unfair suddenly to tell those who have been counting on the current system that they *must* stay in longer.

Instead, perhaps the pensionable age could be tied to the average life span, and very gradual increases tied to the prospect of a longer life. The age when the average person retires might also be raised by making more jobs and more training available and by providing better incentives to remain in the work force, such as an increase in the currently minimal bonus paid to those who postpone retirement until after age 65, and liberalization of the retirement income test. Other methods involving the postponement of retirement in return for "time off" for education or leisure are discussed in Chapter 3.

Suggestions offered in the preceding paragraphs cover only some of the improvements which could be made in the Social Security system. As noted earlier, a decision on whether to emphasize private pensions or Social Security can only be properly made after fuller study of the macro-economic impact of the private pension system. In any case the various income systems must be closely orchestrated. Thus the availability of work and the amount of income earned from work, a subject discussed in the next section, should influence the direction which Social Security takes in the future.

OPTIONS FOR POLICIES AFFECTING INCOME FROM WORK AND ALLOCATION OF TIME BETWEEN WORK, LEISURE, AND EDUCATION

Reasons for Retirement. It is evident that people retire for a number of different reasons, and of these, health and mandatory retirement are among the more important. It is also evident that many older persons would prefer some form of work to full retirement. How many is not clear. Statistics in this area should be viewed with a wary eye, because the data can be chosen to make it appear that the lack of job opportunity is either important or unimportant. Statistics from a single survey, the 1974 Harris Poll, illustrate the problems. This survey found that 37 percent of retirees 65 and over were forced to retire, and that 31 percent of those retired or unemployed would like to be working. Of the latter, 57 percent said that they were kept from working by poor health, and only 15 percent indicated that the lack of job opportunities was the reason. Yet when asked how serious was the problem of "not enough job opportunities" for them personally, 25, not 15, percent reported it a serious problem. Perhaps health may have been the most important reason prompting retirement from a given job, but if opportunities for lighter or part-time work had been available, some of those retiring because of health might well have taken other jobs.

IMPORTANCE OF LACK OF OPPORTUNITY.   Any one set of data can be misleading. Much depends on how one phrases the questions, whether housewives are included, the age of the respondent, and whether he or she has retired, etc. Table 10.1 illustrates more of the complexities. Health was reported as the most important reason for retirement for those aged 62 to 64; for those age 65, compulsory retirement was the most significant factor. Note that even in the 62–64 age bracket, compulsory retirement and layoffs were as significant a factor as the desire to retire. (Also note how the types of categories utilized can influence the percentages in any one category.)

There is thus much disagreement about how to interpret available data and the extent to which older people are in fact barred from working by mandatory retirement and lack of job opportunities. Less frequently recognized is the impact of what is available on what is desired. As R. M. Belbin states in Chapter 4:

> We have now passed the era when our assessment of individual preferences concerning work and retirement hinged on simplistic questions about whether or not individuals wanted retirement. People adjust to the inevitable. We now realize that it is much more difficult to assess underlying aspirations which indicate how people would exercise their options if given a greater choice.

The lack of sufficient employment opportunities is of obvious concern to the older person who is actively seeking a job and cannot find one. However this lack also affects those retirees who believe that even if they looked they couldn't find employment. A substantial improvement in the quality of life for many older people could thus be achieved by making more employment opportunities available for those who want them. Although it is the incumbents of society's most attractive and autonomous jobs who seem to be most enthusiastic about continuing to work, at present it is the poorest and perhaps the least skilled elderly who want work most or need to work, as Table 10.2 suggests. Making job opportunities available should be a goal of those interested both in the well-being of the elderly and in reducing the future tax burden.

Priorities for Change. The current high unemployment rate renders this a less attractive proposal than it would be in a time of full employment. More jobs for older people are seen as meaning fewer jobs for others. However, the majority of the American public wants a lower rate, and sees a need for more jobs—not just

Table 10.1 Categories of Responses at the Question, "Please Describe Briefly the Most Important Reason for Leaving Your Last Job," by Age at Entitlement: Nonemployed Men Awarded Retired Worker Benefits, July–December, 1968.

Categories of responses	Total	Age at entitlement			
		Total	62-64		65
			62	63-64	
(Percentages unless otherwise specified)					
Number (in thousands):					
Total	140	101	60	41	39
Reporting on reasons	133	96	58	39	37
Total percent	100	100	100	100	100
Health	45	54	57	48	23
Specific illness or disability	29	34	38	30	14
Accident, injury	2	3	3	2	1
General poor health	14	16	16	16	8

Job related	27	20	19	22	44
Compulsory retirement	12	3	1	7	36
Job discontinued, laid off	11	13	14	12	6
Dissatisfied	4	4	4	4	2
General retirement age[a]	7	5	4	6	14
Eligibility for social security or pension	2	2	2	2	1
Age for retirement	6	[b]	2	4	13
Retirement, wanted to retire[a]	17	17	15	19	16
Changed jobs	1	3	1	1	1
Family or personal	3	3	3	4	1
Miscellaneous	1	1	1	–	–

[a]Includes some who reached compulsory retirement age.
[b]Less than 0.5 percent.
Source: Social Security Administration (1976).

Table 10.2 Attitudes Regarding Interest in Work of Persons 65 and Over Who Are Retired or Unemployed, by Income Category (Percentages)

	Total	Under $3,000	$3,000-$6,999	$7,000-$14,999	$15,000 & over
Would like to work	31	43	31	20	23
Would not like to work	65	54	64	76	74
Not sure	4	3	5	4	3
	100	100	100	100	100

Source: National Council on the Aging (1975). Reprinted from *The Myth and Reality of Aging in America*, a study prepared by Louis Harris and Associates, Inc. for The National Council on Aging, Inc., Washington, DC (c) 1975.

for older people but for the whole work force. It may take experimentation with our economy, its forms of organization, and its rules and incentives, to reduce the rate of unemployment. E. F. Schumacher (1975) and others have suggested ideas which might result in more jobs, improvement in the quality of work, more intelligent use of energy resources, and possibly more community feeling. Whether as a nation we will become interested in such major reform is not clear. Even in the absence of such interest, however, a number of steps may be taken to increase opportunities for older people. Many of these have been suggested in the chapters by Morrison and Belbin. My own priority list would include the following:

1. Institutional and economic barriers to part-time employment should be reduced, and incentives to split up jobs or create new part-time jobs should be explored. The Council of Europe recently passed a resolution in support of gradual retirement policies

   designed to avoid the traumatic situation where occupational activity is suddenly stopped, representing an alienating factor for the elderly worker who is suddenly cast out, after a life of activity, into a situation of forcible passivity without any transition whatever (Marziale, 1976, p. 286).

   The Council suggested that gradual retirement for older workers should be linked with the progressive entry of young workers into occupational life, an idea which is worthy of exploration in the U.S. as well.

2. Public service jobs (particularly human service jobs) with decent salaries and opportunities for recognition and advancement should be made more available on a full-time, part-time, or job-shared basis.

3. Job retraining programs could be expanded, with special attention to retraining older workers. Vocational and second career counseling could be made available.

4. Unions might consider shifting their emphasis and beginning to press industry to create lighter or part-time jobs and transitional retirement. Provisions of pension plans requiring mandatory retirement might be modified. Longer vaca-

tions or sabbaticals (in which the United Auto Workers has already expressed interest) might also be sought.

5. The government might set up a model by creating a transitional retirement program, offering part-time jobs, counseling, job retraining, and transfer opportunities to older workers who do not want full retirement. Transitional retirement could begin at any age from 60 to 70, depending on the health and inclination of the worker. Partial pensions rather than the present earnings limitation rule might be a more positive way of encouraging gradual retirement.

A Life Cycle Planning Proposal for the U.S. The life span of the average American citizen has been increasingly compartmentalized into periods devoted first to education, then to work, and then to leisure. The cumulative effect of social legislation over the last 50 years has been to treat education, work and retirement as sequential, isolated activities. Gradually, people are beginning to object to this compartmentalization. One of the first persons to focus upon the issue was Dr. Juanita Kreps, who, by the early 60s, was questioning the policy of "solving" the problem of uneven labor supply and demand not by reducing working hours per week or increasing the length of vacation, but simply by increasing the time spent in retirement (Kreps, 1963). Compartmentalization has also been questioned by educators, who have for some time been discussing "life cycle planning" and have managed to insert a "life-long education" section into the Education Amendments of 1976 (P. L. 94–482). Another sign of this interest was the April 1977 National Conference on Life Cycle Planning, in which a number of Senators and corporation leaders participated.

Thus far, however, little research or policy planning has been done on how to implement broad proposals calling for more flexible allocation of work, leisure, and education. To begin, we might do well to find out how the French system of taxing employers to provide paid leave for education and training is working out in practice. There are other areas for study here in the U.S. Some of our major corporations already offer generous provisions for educational and public service leave. What are the benefits to the companies, and what are the costs and drawbacks?

Research in these areas might suggest whether government incentives for other companies to follow suit are desirable (or necessary). Research is also needed on employee preferences and on existing experiments providing for part-time work by older employees, shared work and/or apprentice programs, retraining programs, etc.

Such research should be useful in helping to formulate and evaluate proposals for change, including the following life cycle planning proposal, which combines elements of proposals suggested by Jule Sugarman, Gosta Rehn, and Malcolm Morrison (Chapter 3). The proposal would offer each adult either or both of the following options.

The Reallocation Option.

1. Under this option, every working person would accrue credits toward government sabbatical stipends administered as part of the Social Security system. Each person would be granted three years' worth of credits. The stipend would provide a salary replacement so that the individual could leave his or her job to undertake further education, retrain for another job, do volunteer work, or simply go fishing. The three years could be taken in one-year chunks at any point during the lifetime.

2. Those who utilized their credits would forego the normal eligibility for full Social Security retirement benefits at age 65 (or early retirement at 62). Instead, to receive their Social Security they would be required to work (full or part-time) beyond the normal benefit age, to make up for time off taken earlier. They would be excused from this requirement only because of poor health, in which case they would receive disability rather than retirement benefits.

3. Some limitation might have to be imposed on the number who could use their credits in any one year. Either a lottery or a first-come, first-served system might suffice. Additionally, a person would be required to work for at least eight years before utilizing any credits.

4. The present age discrimination law would have to be modified to forbid firing a person for reasons of age until at least age 70 (rather than age 65, as the law now stands).

5. Employers would be encouraged to provide full or part-time jobs for people over 60 through some form of tax relief, possibly the waiver of Social Security taxes for employees above the age of 60.

The Sabbatical Option.

1. Under this option (which would differ very little from voluntary saving) a person would be able to pay a set percentage of his salary or wages into a government fund. At the end of a specified period (probably seven to ten years), the worker would get the money back, plus interest, and thus be allowed a year's sabbatical. The advantage to the individual would be that the government not only would guarantee a set rate of interest (probably five to six percent), but would index his account to keep up with inflation in addition to paying the set interest rate. No strings would be attached to the use made of the sabbatical year. Unlike Sugarman's plan, this one would be voluntary.

2. Unions could negotiate with employers for guarantees that at the end of each sabbatical, employees could return to the same or an equivalent job. Employees not protected by unions would have to negotiate their own arrangements in advance. They might utilize written contracts, which would guarantee jobs except in cases of bankruptcy or specified economic reverses of the guaranteeing firm. (Such contracts could be used in the reallocation option as well.)

The reallocation option proposal has certain drawbacks. The biggest one is the possibility that too many people would decide to avail themselves of their reallocation credits within a short period of time and thus cause both a labor shortage and a drain on the public treasury. This problem could be avoided by imposing a limitation on the number who could use the credits in any year. Another problem is that some of the people who used the credits would not be able to work past 65 because of ill health (or death), and thus the system would cost more than a straight trade-off of work past normal retirement age and non-work at earlier ages. Therefore, funds from general revenue taxation as well as payroll taxes should be used to support the system.

PROSPECTS

The term "golden age" is more often used ironically than seriously in this country, reflecting our understanding that for many people, old age is not a good age. Too many needs—for roles and respect as well as income—are still unmet. A number of social changes could be made at no expense to our pocketbooks. But the price tag on Social Security, pensions and government service programs is high, and will increase. Can we afford the cost of meeting the income and income-in-kind needs of a growing older population?

Before we react to the cost implications of demographic projections by freezing Social Security, welfare, medical or home health benefits, we ought to examine a number of factors outlined in this book. For example, the increased numbers of elderly probably will be largely counterbalanced by decreased numbers of children, with the result that overall dependency costs will not rise very much. Furthermore, some elderly are well off and could be taxed more heavily by such means as including Social Security benefits as taxable income. Disproportionately generous state, local and military pensions can be pared back, and a cap can be placed on total benefits received by double dippers. Financial incentives for early retirement can be eliminated. Of greatest potential, however, is the option of creating more opportunity and incentive for older people to remain in the work force, thus substantially reducing Social Security and pension costs.

Barring either a serious economic crisis or a breakthrough in prolonging life, it seems clear that we *can* afford to sustain and, where needed, increase the income of the elderly. How easily we can do so will depend on how well we manage our national economy.

However, adequate income alone does not in itself guarantee a good old age, as Robert Butler (1975), Sharon Curtin (1972), and Alex Comfort (1976) have shown so forcefully. Most Americans realize we still need to improve the quality of old age. What we have not fully appreciated is the impact of one phase of life on another. The quality of middle age—whether one learns to enjoy leisure, or has opportunities for education and retraining —affects the quality of old age and indeed, whether one survives to old age. Conversely, the *prospective* quality of old age colors the quality of middle age. If one could count on a decent income and good health care, and could foresee continued chances for work and education as well as leisure, then the prospect of growing old —so dreaded by many Americans—might appear much brighter.

REFERENCES

Anderson, O. W. Reflections on the sick aged and the helping systems. In B. L. Neugarten, & R. J. Havighurst (Eds.), *Social policy, social ethics, and the aging society.* Washington, D.C.: U.S. Government Printing Office, 1976.

Ball, R. M. Income security after retirement. In B. L. Neugarten, & R. J. Havighurst (Eds.) *Social policy, social ethics, and the aging society.* Washington, D.C.: U.S. Government Printing Office, 1976.

Brotman, H. B. Income and poverty in the older population in 1975. *The Gerontologist,* 1977, *17*(1), 23–26.

Butler, R. N. *Why survive? Being old in America.* New York: Harper & Row, 1975.

Burns, E. Social Security in Evolution. *Social Service Review,* 1965, *39,* 129–140.

Comfort, A. *A good age.* New York: Crown, 1976.

Congressional Budget Office. *Poverty status of families under alternative definitions of income.* Background paper No. 17. Washington, D.C.: U.S. Government Printing Office, January 13, 1977.

Curtin, S. R. *Nobody ever died of old age.* Boston: Little, Brown & Co., 1972.

Drucker, P. *The unseen revolution: How pension fund socialism came to America.* New York: Harper & Row, 1976.

Elwood, P. M., Jr. Models for organizing health services. In I. K. Zola, & J. B. McKinlay (Eds.) *Organizational issues in the delivery of health services.* New York: Prodist, 1974.

Haneberg, R. L. Focus on ERISA: Present problems, future concerns. *Pension World,* 1977, *13*(2), 41–48.

Harris, L. & Assoc. *The myth and reality of aging in America.* Washington, D.C.: The National Council on The Aging, 1975.

Henry, J. How pension fund socialism didn't come to America. *Working Papers for a New Society,* 1977, *4*(4), 78–87.

Kreps, J. (Ed.). *Employment, income and retirement problems of the aged.* Durham, N.C.: Duke University Press, 1963.

Kreps, J. *Lifetime allocation of work and income.* Durham, N.C.: Duke University Press, 1971.

Lovins, A. B. Emergy strategy: The road not taken? *Foreign Affairs,* 1976, *55*(1), 66–96.

Maddox, G. L. Community and home care: The unrealized potential of an old idea. Address delivered to the Anglo-American Conference on the Elderly, May 18, 1976.

Marziale, F. Resolution of the Council of Europe on social security measures to be taken in favour of pensioners and persons remaining in activity after pensionable age. *International Social Security Review,* 1976, *29*(3), 284–289.

Okun, A. M. *Equality and efficiency: The big tradeoff.* Washington, D.C.: The Brookings Institution, 1975.

Rosenfeld, A. *Prolongevity.* New York: Alfred A. Knopf, 1976.

Schumacher, E. F. *Small is beautiful: Economics as if people mattered.* New York: Harper & Row, 1975.

Schulz, J. H. *The economics of aging.* Belmont, California: Wadsworth Publishing Co., 1976.

Schulz, J. H. Public Policy and the Future Roles of Public and Private Pensions. In G. S. Tolley and R. V. Burkhouser (Eds.) *Income Support Policies for the Aged.* Cambridge, Mass.: Ballinger, 1977.

U.S. Department of Health, Education and Welfare. *Elderly Widows.* Statistical Memo No. 33, (OHD) 77-20015. Washington, D.C.: U.S. Government Printing Office, 1976.

U.S. Department of Health, Education and Welfare. *Income and Poverty Among the Elderly: 1975. Statistical Reports on Older Americans.* Washington, D.C.: U.S. Government Printing Office, 1977.

U.S. Department of Health, Education and Welfare, Social Security Administration. *Reaching retirement age. Findings from a survey of newly entitled workers, 1918–1970.* Washington, D.C.: U.S. Government Printing Office, 1976.

U.S. Department of Labor. Bureau of Labor Statistics. Three budgets for a retired couple. *News,* August 19, 1976.

U.S. Senate, Committee on the Budget. *Tax expenditures. Compendium of Background Material on Individual Provisions,* 94th Congress, 2nd Session. Washington, D.C.: U.S. Government Printing Office, 1976.

U.S. Senate, Special Committee on Aging. *Developments in aging: 1975 and January–May 1976* (Report No. 94–998), Part 1. 94th Congress, 2nd Session. Washington, D.C.: U.S. Government Printing Office, 1976.

U.S. Senate, Special Committee on Aging. *Developments in Aging: 1976.* Part 1. Report No. 95–88, 95th Congress, 1st Session. Washington, D.C.: U.S. Government Printing Office, 1977.

INDEX